Praise for Pamela Peeke and *Fight Fat After Forty*

"Another piece of the stress management puzzle is yet better defined! Dr. Peeke explores how stress directly affects your body composition and shows how you can control your weight by harnessing the mind's power to achieve stress resilience."
—Herbert Benson, M.D., Mind-Body Medical Institute, Associate Professor of Medicine, Harvard University, author of *The Relaxation Response* and *Timeless Healing*

"Dr. Pam Peeke, a wizard of science, medicine, and the tender mysteries of the human heart, shows us how to shed the physical and mental weight that prevents us from becoming most fully and vibrantly ourselves."
—Joan Borysenko, Ph.D., author of *Minding the Body, Mending the Mind*

"In *Fight Fat After Forty*, Dr. Peeke has made critical contributions as to how stress influences obesity and why obesity so often defeats the efforts of the most motivated dieters. She is the ideal person to be teaching the interested nonscientist about this important subject."
—Robert Sapolsky, Professor of Biological Sciences, Stanford University School of Medicine, and author of *Why Zebras Don't Get Ulcers*

"This book isn't about middle-aged spread, it's about how stress makes you fat. . . . This book has far more brainpower than most diet books . . . [its] value is largely in its explanation of the science and its charty tools intended to help you change when and how you eat—and react to stress."
—*The Washington Post*

ABOUT THE AUTHOR

Pamela Peeke, M.D., M.P.H., devoted three years to investigating the link between stress and fat at the National Institutes of Health as a senior research fellow. She is an internationally recognized expert and speaker in the fields of nutrition and stress as well as the newly evolving field of integrative medicine. She regularly appears as a science and health news commentator for the major networks. She is Assistant Clinical Professor of Medicine at the University of Maryland School of Medicine.

Fight **Fat** After Forty

The Revolutionary Three-
Pronged Approach That Will
Break Your Stress-Fat Cycle
and Make You Healthy, Fit, and
Trim for Life

Pamela Peeke,
M.D., M.P.H.

PENGUIN BOOKS

PENGUIN BOOKS
Published by the Penguin Group
Penguin Putnam Inc., 375 Hudson Street,
New York, New York 10014, U.S.A.
Penguin Books Ltd, 27 Wrights Lane, London W8 5TZ, England
Penguin Books Australia Ltd, Ringwood, Victoria, Australia
Penguin Books Canada Ltd, 10 Alcorn Avenue,
Toronto, Ontario, Canada M4V 3B2
Penguin Books (N.Z.) Ltd, 182-190 Wairau Road,
Auckland 10, New Zealand

Penguin Books Ltd, Registered Offices: Harmondsworth, Middlesex, England

First published in the United States of America by
Viking Penguin, a member of Penguin Putnam, Inc., 2000
Published in Penguin Books 2001

2 3 4 5 6 7 8 9 10

A NOTE TO THE READER
This book is not intended as a substitute for the medical recommendations of
physicians or other health-care providers. It reflects the author's experiences, studies,
research, and opinions. Neither the author nor the publisher shall be liable or
responsible for any health, welfare, or subsequent damage allegedly arising
from the use of any information contained in this book.

"Glycemic Index of Common Food Sources of Carbohydrate" by
Jennifer C. Brand-Miller, appeared in American Journal of Clinical Nutrition,
October 1995, 62(4). Used with permission

"Rockport Walking Chart" reprinted by permission of The Rockport Company, Inc.

THE LIBRARY OF CONGRESS HAS CATALOGED THE HARDCOVER EDITION AS FOLLOWS:
Peeke, Pamela.
Fight fat after forty : the revolutionary three-pronged approach that will break
your stress-fat cycle and make you healthy, fit, and trim for life / Pamela Peeke.
p. cm.
ISBN 0-670-88919-9 (hc.)
ISBN 0 14 10.0181 X (pbk.)
1. Middle-aged women—Health and hygiene. 2. Stress management.
3. Weight loss. I. Title.
RA778.P317 2000
613.7'045—dc21 99–054167

Printed in the United States of America
Set in Sabon
Designed by Jaye Zimet

I dedicate this book to all of the women and men who have shared their life stories with me. I will never cease to be amazed at the courage, tenacity, and depth of passion they have shown as, together, we continue to find ways to live more joyfully.

Specifically, I want to dedicate this book to my patients who have tirelessly given of their time and effort to help me understand their life journeys. They have taken part in retreats, focus groups, and gatherings to share their histories and experiences as they have grappled with the issues of self-esteem, accomplishment, self-care, and self-worth in the face of the constant onslaught of life's daily stresses.

Some of their stories are told in this book—Naomi, Marcia, Marg, Karen, Madelyn, Helen, Eileen, Johari, Gioia, Deb, Jane, Susan, Barbara, Sylvia, Hillary, and so many others. I want to especially mention Leslie Milk, without whom this book would have been impossible. I will never be able to thank her enough for her wit and insights about how truly powerful women are.

My greatest reward for my professional work is spending time with these extraordinary people. They are my muses.

"Life is largely a process of adaptation to the circumstances in which we exist. A perennial give-and-take has been going on between living matter and its inanimate surroundings, between one living being and another, ever since the dawn of life in the prehistoric oceans. The secret of health and happiness lies in successful adjustment to the ever-changing conditions on this globe; the penalties for failure in this great process of adaptation are disease and unhappiness."

—Hans Selye, M.D.
The Stress of Life

Foreword

I first spoke to Dr. Pamela Peeke almost a decade ago. The call was from the University of California at Davis, where she was completing her work as a Pew Foundation Scholar at their famed graduate school of nutrition.

Her voice was clear and strong, and what she wanted from me was unequivocal. "I have been following your work on stress science for years and I would like to work with you," she told me in her usual direct fashion. During that initial discussion, I realized she was a physician with a clear and determined purpose in life: to make a difference. A few months later she and her immense energy were in my laboratory at the National Institutes of Health, conducting exciting new research studies showing the connection between stress and weight.

My research at the time was focused on improving our understanding of how stress hormones influence the mind and body during human development and women's life transitions from birth through menopause. Dr. Peeke's work enriched my laboratory's scope and widened my own perspective in a field that I had only lightly touched in my past research. It did not take us long to realize that stress and the hormones secreted during stress are major culprits in the development of obesity. And furthermore, that stress management, based on solid scientific evidence, could make a life-saving difference in reversing what appears to be a national epidemic of weight gain, especially after the age of forty.

Over the past twenty years, scientists progressively realized that not all fat in the body is a cause of illness. It appeared that the most life-threatening fat was not the excess weight on hips and thighs, but the fat situated deep inside our abdomens. Normally, this intra-abdominal, or visceral fat, is there to help provide the calories or fuel needed in times of physical stress. Dr. Peeke and I refer to this fat as "stress fat." It was already known that unhealthy eating and physical inactivity caused more stress fat to accumulate. Research soon revealed that chronic, uncontrolled stress could also result in excess stress fat, even if that individual was not overweight. And that the excess fat was potentially lethal, causing metabolic abnormalities, high blood pressure, diabetes, and heart disease. The body weight associated with this type of fat should then be referred to as Toxic Weight.

Furthermore, although the accumulation of Toxic Weight can actually start in the womb, individuals over the age of forty are at particular risk for this type of weight gain. Of great concern are over-forty women as they journey through the perimenopause. Hormonal changes, increasing stresses of caregiving as well as difficulty setting priorities for their own self-care are the triple threat that leads to the accumulation of Toxic Weight.

Dr. Peeke recognized this situation as a call to arms to make women and men aware of this vicious stress-induced weight-gain cycle. With passion, she has written a state of the art book, explaining in simple terms the complex science behind the stress-fat connection and what can be done to reverse it.

As her scientific mentor, it was a great pleasure to meet and speak with many of her patients whose life stories are included and analyzed in this book and to see the results of Dr. Peeke's therapeutic approach with them. I understand that it takes more than research, more than science, more than a technician in a white coat to make a difference. It takes someone special to bring that knowledge out of the laboratory and into the hands of women and men who need it. Using a holistic, well-integrated approach, combining science with practical tools to cope with daily stresses, Dr. Peeke provides a rational guide to sustainable lifestyle changes that will finally break the stress-fat cycle for life.

—George P. Chrousos, M.D., Endocrinologist, Bethesda, Maryland

Acknowledgments

In December 1998, *Shape* magazine published an article entitled "When Stress Makes You Fat." In it, I had explained for the first time in a consumer publication the basic science behind the stress-fat connection. This was followed by a television appearance and then a tidal wave of telephone calls from the media. I had apparently hit a nerve. Two of those phone calls came from people who would eventually become pivotal players in the conception and final writing of this book. First, I thank Amanda Urban at International Creative Management for her relentlessness in tracking me down and convincing me that now was the time to write my book. I am deeply grateful for her leadership and direction and for mentoring me as my literary agent.

Second, synchronicity was in action when quickly following Amanda's phone call Molly Stern was on the line. Molly, who became my editor at Viking, had also read the article and seen the TV morning show and knew the book was a must. I cannot express in words my eternal gratitude for her diligence and dedication to the successful completion of this book. With eternal patience, she walked me through this journey, teaching me the whys and wherefores as we painstakingly designed and developed the concepts together. Her joyful humor and wit were my stress neutralizers as the book evolved. Amanda and Molly guided me through some of my toughest challenges, as this book was a journey on so many levels. For them, I cannot express enough thanks.

When I first met George Chrousos, M.D., at the National Institutes of Health, I knew instantly that he would become one of the most important mentors of my professional life. A soft-spoken, handsome Greek academician, he welcomed me into his laboratory with an open mind and heart and provided me with every opportunity to explore the world of stress physiology, a field of research in which he is one of the world's most respected scientists. He was a patient teacher whose major goal was always the pursuit of truth, no matter how late we worked into the night or through the weekends. My real joy is continuing my work with him piecing together the puzzles we create by our own discoveries. This book would have been impossible without his knowledge and guidance, and for that I am eternally grateful.

Mary Supley and Sharon Frishett were the core of the research and writing team. Without these two energetic and indefatigable young women, this book could not have happened. Nancy Turner, my trusty assistant, was by my side throughout, always asking what more she could do.

I want to thank Ida-Marie LaQuatra, R.D., Ph.D., for her invaluable input with all of the nutrition research and program development. Adrienne Ressler was our body image expert. Also, Elena Rover, senior health editor for *Ladies' Home Journal,* provided expertise and up-to-date physical activity training exercises and techniques designed specifically for the over-forty woman's body. I thank Stephanie Mansfield for setting the pace with her expert writing skills.

Over time, I found that I relied upon my buddies to help me realize this was all possible. The insatiable wit and humor of Loretta LaRoche, my dear friend, was positively life-saving. Her expertise as one of the leading experts on health and humor was personally therapeutic and helped me see the big picture when all I saw was my computer screen.

I spent hours discussing the plight of fat and fitness with one of my closest friends and colleagues, Barbara Moore, Ph.D., president of Shape Up America! A brilliant scientist and spokesperson for health and nutrition, Dr. Moore continually kept me on my intellectual feet, always pushing me to see further than I thought possible.

When I was a postdoctoral fellow at the University of California at Davis, I studied under one of this country's great minds in nutrition science, Judith Stern, Sc.D. Since that time, she has become a wonderful friend and mentor and her nurturing words kept me on the straight and narrow.

As I wrote this book, I received advice and counsel from so many scientists and colleagues in the field of stress. Their words of encouragement and wisdom are deeply appreciated. They include Philip Gold, M.D., Chief, Neuroendocrinology Branch, National Institute of Mental Health; Vivian Pinn, M.D., Director of the Office of Research on Women's Health at the National Institutes of Health; Stanford's Robert Sapolsky, Ph.D., and Kenneth Pelletier, M.D., Ph.D.; Robert Lash, M.D., from the University of Michigan; and Herbert Benson, M.D., Director of the Harvard Mind/Body Institute. I especially thank Brian Berman, M.D., of the University of Maryland for the opportunity to teach nutrition science and integrative medicine at the medical center. Teaching is my love of life.

I cannot express enough thanks to the wonderful people at *Shape* magazine for inadvertently getting the ball rolling. Kathy Nenneker shares the vision for spreading the word on getting all women, regardless of age, fit and well. Barbara Harris has always inspired me to teach my patients to embrace the outdoors as the greatest natural stress reducer.

Linda Solheim is my best friend and living through this book project made that clear. Scott Bojan, my trainer, kept me strong and fit while my friend Wanda Von Kleist kept me mentally centered.

Finally, I thank my family for their unconditional patience and love. Victor, Karen, and Rebecca are the wind beneath my wings.

Contents

Introduction

Stress can make you frazzled. Stress can make you sick. But did you also know that stress can make you fat? And keep you fat. It's a scientific fact: how you respond to and cope with stress determines your appetite, body composition, and overall fitness level.

After the age of forty, the accrued stresses of a lifetime, declining metabolism, and the inevitable onset of perimenopause begin to take a physical toll on women. If you are over forty, you are currently going through your third metabolic decrease in three decades. Deposits of fat have settled at your waistline, and your energy level is flagging; changing either of these seems impossible.

If you are a woman over forty, your life is especially frenzied (juggling aging parents, career, spouse, teenage children), and your hormones—including your stress hormones—are beginning to flood your body somewhat unpredictably, which can result in mood swings, muscle fatigue, loss of memory, and intense food cravings. These physical and emotional changes can be exacerbated by chronic, long-term stress, or Toxic Stress, which specifically strikes women between the ages of forty and sixty and leads to self-destructive eating behaviors.

When stress hits, various brain chemicals are released to help the body handle its physical response. One of those chemicals is a powerful appetite trigger, which is why, when Toxic Stress is present, so many women find themselves standing mindlessly at the kitchen counter, foraging for food after a long, hard day.

Toxic Stress puts fat on. Developing a stress-resilient lifestyle can take it off.

The only way to successfully fight fat after forty, develop real physical fitness, and make changes that will lead to a healthier lifestyle is to learn to become more resilient in the face of chronic Toxic Stress and break the stress-fat cycle.

Everyone has a different "stress profile" that determines his or her eating response to stress. Over the last seven years, I have treated hundreds of women who were referred to my medical practice by fed-up internists, frustrated psychiatrists, and other colleagues who saw me as a last resort. I have seen Hollywood actresses, an MTV diva, professional athletes, government officials, corporate CEOs, and other extraordinary women trying to balance high-profile careers and families. My diagnosis? Most were stress eaters. They used food as an anesthesia to numb the pain of their chronic stress, some of which they had been dragging through their lives since childhood. Once we identified the source of the stress, the emotional hunger began to subside and healthy eating took its place.

I'm a doctor. But moreover, I'm a woman, a scientist, and a stress physiologist, and one of the few physicians in this country who is trained in nutrition. Because I always integrate the mind and body in my practice, one of my patients dubbed me her personal "nutri-shrink."

I have been successful with women over forty for one reason: I help them manage the stresses in their lives without destroying themselves.

"Fix my body, and I'll feel better," my patients often say when we first meet. That's not the way it works. Instead, my mantra is simple: a beautiful, healthy body emanates from a healthy mind. I help my patients find the courage to stop carrying around their old stresses and anxieties, to stop the stress of diets and deprivation and find balance in their lives. I can help you, too. But you must understand that the help I will provide is not a pill.

I will teach you to acknowledge and honor the needs of your over-forty-year-old body. To rebalance your mind and body. To turn eating from a stressful torment into a nurturing pleasure. To use your body to neutralize the day's stresses. To trade in the unsatisfying "rewards" of stress eating for other, real rewards that are more fulfilling. I will show you how to kick-start your life and help you make lasting changes in your relationships and careers and, finally, come to peace with your body.

The blueprint? Arming yourself with the science of how your over-forty body operates and why your metabolism and hormones are different now than at any other time of your life.

You will learn to make yourself more important than food, to recognize why your years of yo-yo dieting were so self-destructive and why, if you are a woman in your forties, dieting is both mentally and physically toxic. You will learn how to eat again, but this time tasting and savoring, not gulping and overconsuming to anesthetize the day's stress and to curb your guilt and anxiety about paying attention to yourself. This is true for all women, especially those on the cusp of perimenopause and in their forties and fifties. More than 50 million women will be going through menopause in the next several years. And we have so much in common. We are the women who first went on "the pill," first read *Our Bodies, Ourselves*. Now we are entering another era together.

Women must become aware of certain facts—such as that after the age of forty, the rules of self-care change. For instance, you cannot eat the way you did when you were twenty. In fact, if you have continued to consume the same amount of calories as you did when you were twenty until the age of forty-five, you can expect to be at least thirty to fifty pounds heavier and at risk for health problems.

That fat accumulates around the waist. It is normal to have some fat inside your abdomen. I call this Stress Fat since it is the main source of fat that gives you energy to fight or take flight during stress. Toxic Stress in your life actually causes the deposition of too much of this fat. Too much Stress Fat is dangerous since it places a woman at high risk of heart disease, high blood pressure, high cholesterol, stroke, and diabetes, as well as cancer. I call excess Stress Fat "Toxic Weight." And the primary source of Toxic Weight is Toxic Stress.

Therefore, it's not just a question of whether you can still fit into a little black dress or not; after the age of forty, an expanding waistline can be a serious threat to a woman's health. A recent report published by the National Institutes of Health concluded that a woman whose waist measures thirty-five inches or greater is at great risk of early disease and death. This is the first manual that will help you understand how Toxic Stress put on your fat and what you can do about it.

To understand what happens to your body after forty, you must understand how menopause, as well as chronic stress, affects your body composition. Both of them determine your lean body mass (muscle), bone, and fat accumulation. Achieving physical fitness through regular exercise helps maintain optimal body composition. I always tell my patients that "fit" looks and feels better than "thin."

Fit bodies fit into clothes better. Furthermore, fit bodies can fit into smaller sizes at higher weights because their greater percentage of muscle mass reconstructs the body to a more compact, firmer body shape.

I define health simply as successful adaptation to life. To achieve this goal, it is important to maintain a balance of physical and mental fitness—which is what my patients have learned. I will help you understand:

- **How to live a stress-resilient lifestyle**
- **How to keep your stress hormones in check**
- **How to trim your waist of Toxic Weight**
- **How weight loss is possible based on understanding your individual "Stress Profile"**
- **How to jump-start your metabolism**
- **How to regain lost muscle mass after forty**
- **Why diets don't work—but good eating will**
- **How to curb stress-appetite cravings**

There is real science behind all this, but I don't want you to be intimidated. I have tried to translate the research into an easily understood manual for every woman that I hope will become an important guidebook in the years ahead. A balance of mind and body fitness sustained for life is our goal. Be patient. When I ask my patients who are anxious for instant results to name one thing of value in their lives that happened overnight or by taking shortcuts or cutting corners, they can't think of anything.

I have developed three templates that will provide you the tools to fight fat after forty. Consider them to be the spokes of a wheel, the hub of which is the achievement of Stress Resilience.

The first template involves learning to develop a Stress-Resilient personality. My tactics are based on research by and theories of mind/body experts as well as my own clinical experience. You will learn to adapt to the stresses of life and care for yourself at the same time you care for others. You will learn how to make the transition between the more routine, peaceful times of your life (Plan A) and the more challenging ones (Plan B). In the first template, I refer to this as regrouping. I believe that those who can learn to regroup and make appropriate transitions throughout life without self-destruction are the most successful at adapting to stress.

The second template focuses on learning how to destress your eating and use food to keep your stress hormones in check. I will show you how to successfully navigate the most dangerous time of the day for stress eating—midafternoon to evening—and how to plan and prepare for, as well as accommodate, your menopausal metabolism. You will learn how to distinguish between hunger ("I need to survive") and stress-induced appetite ("I want to numb stress"). You will also learn how to taste and savor your favorite foods, not just gulp them down.

The third template teaches you how to incorporate a variety of stress-reducing physical activities into your daily routine. You will be amazed at the immediate improvement in your energy level, and, at the same time, you will notice that your Stress Resilience is increasing.

Finally, my patients will share with you their secrets of success in learning how to regroup and stay on track when everything doesn't go according to plan. Their words of wisdom will be your comfort and guide as you begin your journey. Throughout this book, you will hear the voices of my patients as they share their own life journeys. You may identify with their pain as well as their joy, and I hope you will find their stories inspiring.

This is the second half of your life. You have the power to make your future years rich and rewarding. This book will show you that how we cope with life's challenges determines whether we will maintain control over our bodies as we age.

So many women have sat across from me, saying "Dr. Peeke, I don't understand what is happening to me."

The first thing I tell them is "You're not alone."

Part I
Stress Put On the Fat

The Stages
of Stress

■ The Early History of Stress

I spend quite a bit of time in airports between flights, and I've found through the years that I've spent much of my waiting time watching for at least one traveler to implode. It almost always happens. Did you ever notice that?

Whether people are jostling for position at the baggage claim or fighting for a taxi, their nerves are frazzled and frayed. Airports are the perfect stress science laboratory.

One of my most memorable episodes happened when a flight I was about to take was inexplicably canceled. Along with a throng of other passengers, I was herded from one concourse to another and not given any information on the next available flight. Finally, we were told to go to a certain gate, where we would be issued a new boarding pass. I got my aerobic activity walking from one end of the airport to the other—and, of course, my resistance training carting what felt like fifty pounds of luggage.

When I finally huffed up to the gate, I joined the long line of unhappy passengers. The ticket agent behind the desk was desperately trying to do what he could. One man, about third in line, was tapping his foot anxiously. He had the Armani suit. He had the cell phone. He had the designer leather briefcase. And he was not happy. I could see, even from the back, that he was the one, the Imploder.

I waited. I watched. Sure enough, eventually he just couldn't handle it anymore. You could tell he was getting more and more stressed out. He abruptly stepped out of line, pointed at the young ticket agent, and yelled, "Do you *know who I am*?"

You could have heard a pin drop in the boarding area. I thought, "Oh, no, we're going to have a fight!"

Without missing a beat, the ticket agent calmly looked up at the man standing in front of the Imploder and said, "Sir, could you please help me? I would like you to assist the man behind you. He doesn't seem to *know who he is*!"

Needless to say, the Imploder was more than a little upset. He made a fuss about seeing the "supervisor," but then, red-faced, he took his boarding pass and sat down.

When I finally got up to the counter, I couldn't help but ask the young agent how he had managed that confrontation so gracefully. "Have you spent seven years in Tibet?" I asked with a laugh.

"No," he answered. "Come on, think of what I do for a living. Most of my customers are anxious and in a hurry." He used calm humor to neutralize a highly charged situation. He had a plan that worked for him.

I realized this is what life is all about: developing a plan that works. After learning what stress does to the human body, you'll be able to develop a plan that works for you.

Hans Selye, M.D., the father of stress physiology, said, "Life is stress and stress is life." But for many years, most advice on how to handle stress was within the purview of the science of psychology. Magazine articles, which ofttimes recommended that you "chill out . . . calm down . . . take a deep breath," rarely mentioned the scientific basis for those suggestions. We now have better science to help clarify the issue. I'm going to show you the irrefutable and elegant science behind stress and how to manage it.

Ironically, our understanding of the effects of stress began with a promising young scientist—Selye—in 1936. Originally, he wasn't interested in studying stress. Instead, he did research in the field of reproductive medicine, specifically the function of the ovaries. Assisting another colleague, he worked with rats in a lab, tagging them and observing their behavior. When they had lived out their natural lives, Selye would perform an autopsy on each of them to examine their ovaries.

In the laboratory, Selye tried frantically to tag the rats without dropping them. I don't know if you've ever tried to pick up rats, but they don't like it very much. Selye spent much of his time chasing the rats after inadvertently dropping them. Later, when performing autopsies on the rats, he made a startling discovery. To his amazement, the rats he had repeatedly dropped all had ulcers whereas the others did not.

At first he was unsure of what this discovery meant. He thought there might be a relationship between the stress of the dropping—a mental function—and its effects on body systems—the ulcers. In other words, what occurred in the mind affected the body. To prove his point, Selye decided to do a second study. This time, he studied two groups of rats. One group was treated normally, lived well, ate well, and was basically left alone. The other group he routinely dropped on schedule, every day. It may seem like a strange experiment, but scientific investigations are often that way. Many times, great discoveries occur through serendipity.

When the second group of rats finally died, Selye found ulcers in almost all of them. He had proven to himself that there was a direct relationship between mental stress and bodily disease.

Over the past twenty years, many scientists have devoted their careers to studying the effects of psychological stress on the body. For instance, Tiffany Fields, Ph.D., at the University of Miami School of Medicine, published studies that showed that therapeutic massage could accelerate the rate of growth of premature infants. Such babies endure tremendous physical and psychological stress. Hands-on nurturing was able to neutralize growth inhibition normally caused by their high level of chronic stress.

Judging from the discoveries by Selye, Fields, and others, it seems we need frequent caressing or nurturing to reverse the effects of chronic stress. Every person perceives stress and handles it in a way that is comfortable to her. Some people are born with the ability to handle stress with greater ease than others. These individuals are actually born with body tissues that are more resistant to stress hormones and, therefore, hardier. Many factors must be considered when trying to understand what it takes to achieve the goal of Stress Resilience in the handling of daily life.

I have always been fascinated with what is required to achieve Stress Resilience. I am particularly interested in the role nutrition plays in improving or worsening daily stress. In pursuit of that goal, I became a Pew Foundation postdoctoral scholar in nutrition and metabolism while at the University of California at Davis. During my studies, it had become clear to me that so much of the disease and death I was observing as a physician was a direct result of how patients dealt with life stresses. It appeared that harboring chronic stress is toxic to most body systems. In addition, uncontrolled, chronic stress seemed to lead to destructive eating, poor nutrition, and a variety of diseases, including heart disease and diabetes. I wanted to understand why chronic stress exerts such a powerful force on the body.

After observing my patients over the years, I realized that everyone needs to be in a balanced state of mind and body. The achievement of this balanced state requires regular physical movement and appropriate eating. My goal was to develop a way of understanding how eating, exercise, and a Stress-Resilient attitude can extend the length and quality of life.

While at the University of California, I became acquainted with one of the leading scientists in the field of stress physiology, George Chrousos, M.D., Chief of the Pediatric Endocrinology Section of the National Institutes of Health (NIH) Developmental Endocrinology Branch. Dr. Chrousos and his team at the NIH had laid down the foundation for the study of the relationship between chronic stress and body systems such as immune function, reproduction, and growth. In 1990, I was invited to join his laboratory to study the relationship between chronic stress and nutrition.

At the same time as I began my work in Chrousos's laboratory, Bernadine Healy, M.D., became the first female director of the NIH. Under her tenure, the NIH Office of Research on Women's Health was founded to promote the study of women's health. Previous to that time, women had rarely been invited to participate in major medical studies. Specifically, women over the age of forty were only infrequently studied and usually only for rare medical conditions. Data on how women over forty aged and what affected that aging process, including chronic stress, were typically not gathered. This new interest in women's health care inspired me to investigate gender-specific responses to stress, which eventually led me to examine how women in the perimenopause handle chronic stress.

As I began my research, Chrousos taught me to appreciate the rich history of stress science, which extends back to the ancient Greeks. The Greeks were well aware of the effects of stress on the human body and referred to calm or balance as "harmony." We now call this harmony "homeostasis," which is derived from the Greek word meaning "steady state." Ancient physicians and philosophers realized that stress is a challenge to this balance. Disturbances to homeostasis are now called "stressors." The ways in which we respond to these stressors are our "adaptive responses." For the purpose of survival, the main function of the adaptive responses is maintaining balance and homeostasis.

As far back as 350 B.C., Hippocrates wrote about "health" as meaning the harmonious balance of mind and body and "disease" as being disharmony. Later, the French scientist Claude Bernard (1813–1878) talked about the stability of the internal landscape and first described the "*milieu intérieur* formed by the circulating organic liquid which surrounds and bathes all the tissue elements." While Bernard did not identify this liquid, we now know that it contains stress hormones that, if triggered on a constant basis, can have harmful effects on the body.

Of course, there are different types of stress and stressors of varying intensity and duration. Getting a speeding ticket is certainly stressful, but not as serious as the death of a loved one, a divorce, or getting a surprise audit by the IRS. But when everyday stress becomes very difficult to manage, a person is left feeling chronically out of control and overwhelmed. This can be an insidious process that results in a constant, dull, ever-present psychological background noise of which one may not even be aware.

The process may begin with a childhood hurt and/or abuse that is then carried into adulthood. It can even begin *in utero* if a pregnancy is stressful.

Research has shown that cortisol can be transferred from a mother to her fetus *in utero*. In essence, jumpy mothers have jumpy babies. Stressed-out mothers expose the fetus's cells to higher than normal levels of stress hormones. More serene mothers tend to have calmer babies. Premature infants are a special case; they are under incredible stress and thus have higher than average levels of stress hormones. This may cause their brains to become more sensitive to stressors. Later in life, they may be at risk to develop emotional problems, such as depression. Their response to stress may most likely fall in the abnormal range.

Research has also shown that many children who had a difficult time *in utero* may go on to become adults who have a stress response to life that is almost always toxic. They become overweight. They may be fragile and unable to absorb and deal with even minor daily annoyances. There is a growing body of research evidence that severe stress early in life has long-term effects on the brain's ability to adapt to stress normally. Trauma or stress in infancy, childhood, or adolescence can cause prolonged hypersensitivity to stress as an adult. People who suffer childhood trauma may be more vulnerable to depression and posttraumatic stress disorder (PTSD) later in life. Animal studies using rats and monkeys have shown that exposure to severe stress early in life results in persistently altered stress responses.

The process may also begin later in life with a traumatic personal stress such as being raped. Whatever its origins, human beings simply were not built to carry around constant disturbances to their homeostasis. When chronic stress is present, we now know through research that it sets off a chain of events that can seriously threaten the body. It appears that a healthy body does indeed start with a healthy mind.

When a frightening situation occurs, the body initiates a primal response to save your life. A burst of adrenaline and the stress hormone cortisol are secreted within the body. Together, these biochemicals activate the body to help us escape danger and prolong our survival. After the initial stressful mental shock, the body returns to its normal state, and the hormones that have flooded the muscles and tissues with important survival messages (stay alert, stay focused, get ready to escape) gradually leave the bloodstream.

But what happens when the stress comes in waves, when it is repeated over and over and never resolved? What happens if the stress hormones continue to wash through the system in high levels, never leaving the blood and tissues? What happens, more precisely, when the physical stress response runs constantly and is never shut down?

My colleague Robert Sapolsky, Ph.D., at Stanford University has written extensively about the links between mind and body in his book *Why Zebras Don't Get Ulcers*. Mammals, he postulates, don't get ulcers because they do not normally harbor chronic stress. That is something we humans do all the time.

Imagine a zebra on the Serengeti Plain. He's grazing with other zebras under a noonday sun, enjoying the sweet grass. Through experience, this zebra knows that there must be a lion out there somewhere. He knows enough not to go near the lion's home territory. Instead, he lives in the moment, enjoying the grass, not stressing about where the lion is and dealing with the problem only if the lion actually appears.

We humans, on the other hand, often make a second career out of wondering where our lions are.

■ Toxic Stress

Our science now shows that a sustained high level of cortisol, which results from chronic, unrelenting stress, can have a dangerous, even life-threatening effect on the body. For this reason, I call uncontrollable, chronic stress "Toxic Stress" because it literally poisons your body, making you more vulnerable to colds and flu, fatigue and infections. Toxic Stress can also impair your memory and concentration. And new evidence shows that it can give you a raging appetite! It appears that one of cortisol's major roles is to help refuel the body after each stress episode. Uncontrolled or Toxic Stress keeps the refueling appetite on, thus inducing stress eating and weight gain.

But this is a unique kind of weight gain. The excess fat weight from Toxic Stress, what I have dubbed "Toxic Weight," settles primarily inside the abdomen and is different from fat anywhere else on the body. Too much fat on your thighs may result in mental pain, but it's not associated with deadly diseases. But Toxic Weight, as we shall soon see, is highly associated with heart disease, diabetes, and cancer.

Some stress is what I call Annoying But Liveable (ABL). This includes standing in line at the airport and negotiating traffic jams. ABL stress is integral to daily life.

Other stress is, in fact, life-threatening. Everyday events that should be seen as ABL may become transformed into Toxic Stress when you fall into the habit of harboring anxiety and worry about daily events and relationships. A given individual may perceive a specific life event as either ABL or life-threatening.

I tell my patients that it's not unlike constantly dragging a huge invisible plastic bag of garbage behind you throughout the day, and each new stress adds to the unpleasant mix. Toxic Stress, therefore, is a burden physically, mentally, and emotionally.

True life-threatening stresses are obvious and serious business. These are the events you perceive as endangering your life. Meeting a mugger in a dark alley who is pointing a gun at your head is a life-threatening stress. People who work in dangerous occupations—for instance, as journalists in a war zone—are often exposed to life-threatening stresses.

For many people, however, certain daily situations, which some would perceive as ABL, may be perceived as life-threatening. If you are deathly afraid of public speaking, being asked to give the graduation address at your alma mater may be perceived by your brain as the equivalent of a life-threatening situation even though someone else might relish the challenge and breeze through it. Giving a presentation at work in front of two hundred executives who will be responsible for your performance evaluation may be perceived as life-threatening, even though it's a normal occurrence in the business world. For a terrified speaker, such an experience feels just as life-threatening as a confrontation with a mugger and may actually induce many of the same biochemical responses as occur when a person faces a gun-toting stranger in a dark alley.

ABL stress can be short- or long-term. For example, you may be in the express line at the grocery store and the man in front of you has twenty-five items and you're in a hurry. Or you may receive the good news that your son has won a place on the state soccer team. The bad news is that you will have to chauffeur him all over the state for the next three years, interrupting your normal weekend self-care and family schedule. These are the kinds of daily stresses we all encounter. Many people can handle these life events without imploding and turning them into Toxic Stress.

Stress becomes toxic only when it begins to poison the system and threaten the natural state of homeostasis on a chronic level. A caregiver with a mother diagnosed with Alzheimer's may start to feel guilty about the time she spends away from home. She may stop taking her daily walks. She may decrease her outside activities and turn down social engagements. Feelings of sadness, worry, and anxiety may start to suffocate any thoughts of self-care. Finally, she may lose her sense of balance and sink into a world of limitless giving, damaging her important relationships and disrupting her family life. If she does not maintain the balance of self-care in her life, her caregiving will become toxic.

Toxic Stress is the greatest threat to balance because it never allows the body to shut down the stress response. According to Selye, "Stress is essentially reflected by the rate of all the wear and tear caused by life." When Toxic Stress becomes a way of life, it may be reflected in something as obvious as one's face. All we need to do is to look at the faces at a funeral: the deeply furrowed brows; the frown lines; the look of worry, fatigue, and dejection. Now imagine what that same stress, that same trauma, on a daily basis would do to the delicate tissues inside the body.

When Toxic Stress is allowed to permeate your daily existence, it can result in self-destructive behaviors. These behaviors include anything perceived as an antidote to emotional pain, such as inappropriate eating, excessive alcohol consumption, and use of tobacco or drugs. They can set into motion a downward spiral that only results in more stress. For example, a woman who suffers from Toxic Stress exposes her body tissues to prolonged elevations of cortisol, which, as we have mentioned earlier, induce a stress-response refueling appetite. This may lead to excessive eating and weight gain. The stress eater may then resort to an extreme fad diet to lose her weight, which creates even more Toxic Stress resulting from the food deprivation plus the anxieties and compromised self-worth so characteristic of the diet mind-set. The Toxic Stress of dieting then leads to more weight gain and the accumulation, over time, of Toxic Weight inside the abdomen.

One of my patients, Jennifer, who was at least 50 pounds overweight and in her forties, was shopping for clothes in the maternity department. She first came to see me in 1996. As we discussed her dieting history as a lifelong binge eater, she began confiding in me about her mother, who has always been rail thin and paranoid about her daughter's figure. Jennifer had been put on diet pills at the age of eight. Her mother had also severely restricted her diet, forbidding her even an infrequent snack. In grade school, Jennifer had suffered the humiliation of having to stand in the "fat girl" line at her cafeteria.

Her mother, who had suffered from depression and sought therapy, had been a control freak. Her father had been ineffective and weak. He and Jennifer had been forced to sneak out of the house to eat even a hot dog.

Jennifer wept as she told the story. The memory of that cafeteria line still haunted her. She had been singled out, humiliated, and hurt.

I could have predicted what had happened next: she developed into a binge eater, sneaking forbidden cakes into her closet at night. As soon as she was given an allowance, she secretly spent all her money on junk food and treats. What I could not have predicted was how this childhood stress, once it was revealed to me in my office, would alter the course of Jennifer's life. This was the origin of her problems with food.

The first weeks and months were not easy, as we literally had to reprogram her thinking. But Jennifer bravely took the first steps to reclaim the second half of her life. No longer forced to stand in the "fat girl" line at the school cafeteria, she is now a size 10. How did she do it? By finally processing and learning to neutralize the Toxic Stress of her childhood.

■ Toxic Stress Triggers

Toxic Stress can be triggered by any daily challenge. But my research has shown that there are a few common outside forces that are unique to women over forty. They include:

1. **Childhood traumas**
2. **Perfectionism**
3. **Divorce or change in a relationship**
4. **Caregiving**
5. **Job or career challenges**
6. **Illness, either short-term or chronic**
7. **Dieting**
8. **Menopause**

The greater the chaos in a young girl's life, the greater her propensity to seek an anesthetic to numb the pain later in life. For many, food is the preferred substance. So the seeds of Toxic Stress are often planted during childhood. Eating habits, perception of body image, self-worth, and the response to stress triggers in general are formed in the early years and flourish dangerously after the age of forty.

Johari, a beautiful African-American woman, was forty-three when she first wrote me a letter after reading a magazine article on my work. She was desperate for help. A divorced mother, she weighed more than 200 pounds and had tried every weight loss program without success. She wrote candidly about the childhood experience of so many African-American families who provide rich, fatty foods as the center of most celebrations.

Johari's mother had worked from her home as a caterer, and as a girl Johari would stand at the counter watching her mother prepare tea sandwiches. Since no morsel of food was ever allowed to go to waste, Johari ended up eating the crusts of the bread and the leftover cream cheese fillings. The family's own meals were bountiful—fried catfish, sweet potatoes, gravy—and plates were always cleaned.

As an adult, Johari also learned to use food as a constant source of comfort in times of stress. It became clear that she could not break that pattern of behavior without leaving the psychological shelter of her mother's kitchen. But once she did, she reclaimed the second half of her life, lost 35 pounds, and walked the Marine Corps Marathon!

Perfectionism was Barbara's Toxic Stress trigger. She came to me at thirty-nine years of age, weighing 180 pounds. "Dr. Peeke, I don't know what I'm doing wrong!" she cried. It took several sessions before she began confiding in me about her childhood. She had grown up on a farm, and her younger sister, Marcia, had been extremely overweight. Barbara, on the other hand, had been the beautiful blond cheerleader. But despite her "perfect" Sandra Dee all-American good looks and behavior, she had never felt she was good enough. Smart enough. Pretty enough. Her parents had been emotionally withholding, and the only time her father had ever expressed his love for her was when he was drunk.

Barbara turned to food to numb that pain. She describes her weight gain as the "perfect child's fall from grace." In high school the perfect blond cheerleader ballooned. Then she started crash dieting to regain her "perfect body"—which, of course, was impossible, since crash diets always fail.

She married an emotionally unavailable man (on the surface, "the perfect husband"), gave birth to two kids ("the perfect family"), and ended up deeply depressed. As we began unraveling her history, we found the source of her stress eating: perfectionism triggered by low self-esteem. For her, the greatest pain in life came from her unmet expectations.

I am extremely proud of Barbara. She is still traveling along her journey and still wrestles with stress eating, but she is now running four miles a day and lost 39 pounds in one year.

Divorce is another devastating stress trigger, even if it's a positive move. A traumatic event such as divorce can actually "shut down" a woman's appetite.

My patient Karen, who in her mid-thirties was 75 pounds over-weight, literally stopped eating after her husband left her for another woman. She lost 60 pounds in three months, which I wouldn't rec-ommend to anyone. Of course, once the Toxic Stress subsided, she gained it all back—and more.

Caregiving can also be a serious stress trigger. Marion is a perfect example of how devoting yourself to others can lead to Toxic Stress. Slightly plump while growing up, Marion became the main source of emotional support for her elderly parents and later continued that role in her marriage. She went into a career that also required her to be a "cheerleader" for others, which was, she told me, "totally op-posite of how I felt."

"I would eat to relieve that stress," she said one afternoon, re-counting her endless hours of making sure everyone else in her life was happy. Approaching her forty-fifth birthday, she was desperate for a change. Only when she resolved to balance her caregiving of others with her own self-care did she overcome her stress trigger.

A challenging job or career can be an intense stress trigger. Blind devotion to work can be as dangerous as devotion to others. Naomi, who as a child was the first African-American student in an all-white school district in Washington, D.C., grew up to become extremely ambitious and anxious to overcome all obstacles. This alone would have triggered Toxic Stress. As an adult, she started her own market-ing research firm. She traveled constantly, working hundred-hour weeks. She was under enormous pressure and hadn't taken a vaca-tion in ten years. She came to me wearing a size 16 dress and weigh-ing in the 190s. She was overweight and overwrought. The first thing I did was take my prescription pad and write, "Naomi must take two weeks of vacation every year. No matter what."

She was under Toxic Stress, which she once described to me as being "like a mantle. Like putting on a shawl. It was so present. I needed to do everything right, everything fast. I'm a control freak, and stress is a by-product of that."

Naomi, a reformed stress eater who literally saved her own life, has now achieved a renewed sense of balance in her daily life.

Medical illness can also induce stress. How you handle that stress can either augment healing after the illness or precipitate further deterioration. Learning to manage stress well can save your life.

I recall two patients who had both been diagnosed with Stage I breast cancer. Though the condition generally has an excellent prognosis, both women naturally went into shock at hearing the unsettling news. It was the variation in their response to the news that was so revealing.

The first woman responded by grieving and then regrouping enough to call her doctor and schedule everything that would be necessary to get through the illness: surgery, chemotherapy, radiation. Despite the fact that she was terrified and had no experience with the disease, her response was to take control of the situation. She took immediate action to educate herself and carry through with the best possible treatment.

The second woman was equally terrified. She sat across from me, trembling and in tears, and asked, "Why me?" She was gripped by worry and anxiety. By allowing the disease to define and control her, she became paralyzed and had to struggle to see beyond the diagnosis so she could take the steps necessary to win the battle.

Instead, even though she had a good support system including a husband and friends, she quit her job and stopped doing all the things that had brought her joy. She couldn't sleep, watched TV all day, and overate. Her medical illness turned into Toxic Stress.

Both women faced a life-threatening stress. It was heartening to see one face it so positively, but painful to watch another succumb to the emotional stress.

Stress tends to snowball. Time and again, I have seen the deadly force of the avalanche it can become. And nothing creates Toxic Stress more than voluntary food deprivation.

Dieting is probably one of the most common stress triggers in women over forty. Marcia, Barbara's younger sister, who also grew up on the farm, was extremely overweight as a child. She was teased and taunted and put on diet pills by her mother. By high school, Marcia decided that the best way to lose weight was to stop eating. So she went on a diet: one cup of chicken noodle soup each day. That was it. In college, she lived on cheese, crackers, and green beans and got down to 125 pounds.

She married. After two pregnancies, she was desperate to lose weight and in the early 1990s joined a center that put her a on a high-protein and vegetable diet, with one teaspoon of oil each day. No milk, no grains, no carbohydrates. It didn't take long for her health to break down. Two months later, sick and exhausted, she went to her doctor for a checkup. All of her blood work came back abnormal. She told me during our first visit that it had taken her two years to recover from that crash dieting.

When she first sat in my office, Marcia was at her ideal weight. She appeared fit and trim. I thought, "What's the problem here?" What I couldn't immediately see was that she was traumatized by her anxiety that the fat would return. Despite the fact that she had integrated exercise into her life, eating was still a torment. The Toxic Stress of the years of dieting—including bizarre eating rituals and extreme deprivation—had left her emotionally wounded. A fat head on a fit body was the burden she carried day after day.

Marcia became one of my most challenging patients. My goal was to convince her that she had achieved a healthy weight and fitness level of which she should be proud—and that practicing her healthy mind and body fitness habits daily would allow her to maintain this achievement. Marcia is, therefore, an example of how life-long dieting can result in painful, emotional Toxic Stress.

Most women over forty have "doctorates in dieting," decades of experience compromising their health and eating strangely for the sake of a number on the scale. Whether it's the Grapefruit Diet or cabbage soup, Beverly Hills or Marcia's Miracle One-Cup-of-Chicken-Noodle-Soup-a-Day diet, no one can sustain it for a lifetime. The belief that one can leads to Toxic Stress. For more than thirty years, our generation has been exposed to the idea that dieting is a means to the achievement of personal success and well-being. The tragedy is that all it has fostered is the Toxic Stress of unhealthy lifestyle and body image.

Finally, while busy juggling jobs, families, relationships, medical problems, and personal lifestyle choices, the over-forty woman begins to undergo the last major hormonal transition of her life, the perimenopause. And she has lots of company! By the year 2000, there will be approximately 50 million American women over the age of fifty, about half of whom will have gone through menopause by age fifty-two. Suddenly, coffee break conversations center around shared experiences of memory lapses, mood swings, depression, headaches, insomnia, plummeting libido, irregular periods, and hot flashes. But it's the weight gain that drives most women crazy.

Women in the perimenopause can actually experience a shape shifting. The average weight gain during the five to seven years surrounding the onset of menopause can range from less than 10 to over 25 pounds. And instead of accumulating around the hip and thighs, that weight begins to settle around the waistline. I have heard desperate cries for help from patients who watch with helpless horror as their pants and dresses no longer fit over their expanding abdomen. As one of my patients noted, "I may have been overweight most of my life, but at least I had a waist. Now I feel like I went from an hourglass figure to a shot glass!"

Desperate for a solution, many women once again resort to traditional dieting, only to find that their bodies are less responsive to it. That's because a forty-year-old woman has a very different body than she had ten years earlier. A woman's metabolism traditionally declines at the rate of at least 5 percent per decade of life, starting at the age of twenty. For example, at twenty you may have required 2,000 calories per day to live. By the time you are forty-five, you could require about 300 calories less per day. If you continue to consume the extra calories, you will gain 1 pound every twelve days, or 30 pounds per year. Exercise and careful eating definitely minimize this effect but don't completely erase it.

Declining metabolism and muscle mass, medical disabilities, a decline in physical activity, and an increase in eating out compound the natural changes of the menopausal years. After forty, a woman may find maintaining her self-care to be more difficult, leading to more Toxic Stress. And, as we will show, perimenopausal women are especially vulnerable to carrying their Toxic Stress on their waistline.

2 Science and the Stress Response

■ The Stress Response

Stress keeps us on our toes. It is essential to life. Ideally, we respond to everyday challenges with a positive physical response that is as primal as eating and sleeping. When a threatening event takes place, our bodies are exquisitely designed to swing into action. Every fiber of tissue, every blood cell works in tandem, brain chemicals and hormones pumping messages to our heart, lungs, and limbs. Our stress response was designed to protect us, to save our lives. So how did it become so toxic? What went wrong?

Nothing. We simply became less physical as we got smarter. We invented machines that allowed us to avoid or quickly escape from danger. We no longer have to hunt or forage for our food. Our bodies, once lean, became soft. We substituted intellectual stresses for physical ones. But our primal stress response is *wired* for some sort of physical response. When our ancestors were frightened by something, they physically fought or ran away. That's why the stress response is referred to as the "fight-or-flight" response.

Examine your typical daily stresses: traffic, misbehaving kids, moody husbands, micromanaging bosses, anxious parents, nosy neighbors. Not one single stress requires you to use your body with vigor (run, walk for long distances, climb, lift, fight). Our stress is now all from the neck up. We have evolved into efficiency experts, denying our bodies their natural physical responses to stress. Our world is no longer ruled by predators, and we do not employ our "fight-or-flight" response as originally designed.

But moving our bodies is an essential part of living, and I don't mean you must acquire "buns of steel." I am referring to balancing thought and action. When we don't have a physical release as a way of blowing off stress, it accumulates and may become Toxic Stress.

I will explain, in simple terms, how the stress response operates. Thirty to 40 percent of how we react to stress is genetically defined. To a certain extent, genes from both your mother and your father determine the way you react to stress. The rest of our stress response is learned through life experiences, including life in our mother's uterus. Everyone has different stress triggers, and as we saw earlier, many of these can be dragged from infancy through adolescence and into adulthood.

When the brain first registers a stressful event, it releases a chemical known as corticotropin-releasing hormone (CRH); I call this the "Alarm Hormone." There is always a baseline amount of this hormone in the body, and it can be elevated by anything that stimulates your attention, whether it's fear, excitement, passion, panic, anxiety, happiness, or joy. If the doorbell rings, whether it's the florist holding a dozen roses from an admirer or the mailman with a certified letter from the IRS, the Alarm Hormone, a neurochemical spark directing your attention to the event, will kick in. And once the alarm goes off, it triggers a cascade of neurochemical sparks designed to prepare the body for "fight or flight."

Through an intricate pathway of communications in the brain, the Alarm Hormone then activates the adrenals, two glands located in the abdomen, and tells them to secrete two substances: the "jump-starting" chemical adrenaline (we have all experienced the adrenaline "rush") and the stress hormone cortisol (see Figure 2-1). Cortisol is also known in the scientific literature as a "glucocorticoid," because of its ability to stimulate glucose elevations in our blood and because it is secreted by the outer part of the adrenal gland called the cortex. Together, adrenaline and cortisol activate the body to deal with the stressful event.

Alarm Hormone, cortisol, and adrenaline follow a distinct rhythm of secretion throughout the day. These stress hormones tend

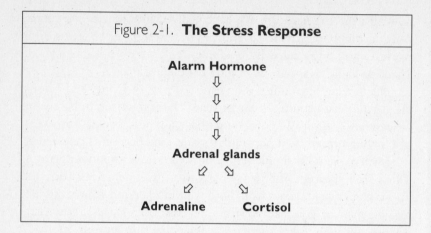

Figure 2-1. **The Stress Response**

Alarm Hormone

Adrenal glands

Adrenaline   **Cortisol**

to peak between 6 and 8 A.M. and begin a gradual decline later in the morning, finally reaching their lowest levels at night. Very gradually, at about 2 A.M., the levels begin to rise again, preparing to awaken you in the morning and help you cope with the next day's stresses (see Figure 2-2).

Within seconds of registering a stressful event, the body is in a state of readiness. It's a chemical version of code red. We are tingling, anxious. Our pupils dilate. Our blood pressure rises. Our thinking and memory improve, our lungs take in more oxygen. Digestion is

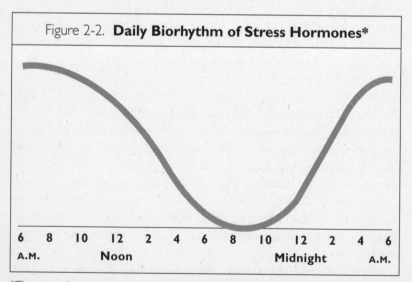

Figure 2-2. **Daily Biorhythm of Stress Hormones***

| 6 | 8 | 10 | 12 | 2 | 4 | 6 | 8 | 10 | 12 | 2 | 4 | 6 |
| A.M. | | | Noon | | | | | | Midnight | | | A.M. |

*The stress hormones are the Alarm Hormone, cortisol, and adrenaline.

momentarily put on hold, allowing the body to concentrate its energy on the muscles needed for the physical stress response. Immune function is momentarily suppressed, diverting all the body's energy to immediate survival. Any sensation of pain is dulled to minimize distraction and focus more attention on the coping mechanism. Every system is on "alert."

Every time the stress response is activated, the Alarm Hormone does more than stimulate the adrenals and the nervous system; it also activates the reward and pain relief areas of the brain. Why do you need to feel reward when you are being stressed? All challenges in life are met with some expectation of achievement. The body is no different. We respond to psychological or physical stressors knowing that their resolution will bring some kind of relief or pleasure.

This is often a learned response. For instance, my patients frequently tell me that it is the pleasure of getting off the treadmill at the end of their morning exercise session that motivates them to go through the healthy physiological stress of the walk. For some the reward of exercising is that it makes you feel marvelous to have it done and over with. It is pleasurable to feel your body tingle with muscular activation and your mind soothed by the calm of accomplishment. After a period of time, you will feel the effects of your body's natural analgesia or pain relief (the runner's high), allowing you to better adapt to the stress.

Most physiological functions in the human body involve stressing the body's systems in a healthy way. For instance, although we do it every day, digesting, metabolizing, and storing food are in fact stressful to the body's systems. Our motivation for carrying out these bodily activities is that the accomplishment of the activity usually yields a pleasurable satiety. If there weren't some pleasure associated with it, some need met, we wouldn't be motivated to eat at all! Fat ingestion seems to be associated with some of the greatest pleasure of all, which is a good thing since fat yields the greatest amount of energy to keep us alive and able to weather life's stresses. To better understand these motivations, researchers genetically altered a mouse and completely removed the reward systems of its brain. What do you think happened to the mouse? With no reward or pleasure associated with any daily bodily actions, it just sat there, no longer motivated by future gain. It had to be fed by tubes because it had absolutely no interest in eating. But though the reward system is an essential motivator of our daily behaviors, in some humans it is dysfunctional. In fact, it is widely held that addictive behavior is associated with a reward system that never creates a feeling of total satisfaction.

The notion of reward will help us understand what can go right as well as wrong in some people's eating patterns under stress, which will be discussed when the stress profiles are described (see Chapter 3).

The "fight-or-flight" response, first described by physiologist Walter Cannon in the early 1900s, is perfect in situations that require you to defend your life or to cope with daily stresses that require

---

Figure 2-3. **Behavioral and Physical Adaptation to Short-term Stress**

Behavioral Adaptations

More:	*Less interested in:*
Aroused	**Eating**
Alert	**Reproduction**
Attentive	**Play**

Physical Adaptations

Increased:
Oxygen and nutrients to stressed site(s), brain, and muscles
Heart rate
Blood pressure
Breathing rate
Fat and carbohydrate available for fuel

Temporarily put on hold:
Growth and reproduction
Digestion
Thyroid function
Pain
Inflammatory response
Immune response

physical strength and endurance. This response is designed to get your body moving away from danger (see Figure 2-5). Cortisol grabs high-octane fat and energy-propelling glucose (carbohydrate) from your body's stores, diverts blood away from temporarily less important organs, such as the stomach and kidneys, and shoots all three to your brain, heart, lungs, and muscles for immediate energy.

Once the immediate stress has passed and you perceive the danger to be over, the adrenaline level in the bloodstream rapidly decreases. Cortisol, on the other hand, lingers in the system and is designed to help bring everything back into balance, to return the body to its natural state of homeostasis. Cortisol actually "turns down" the Alarm Hormone to its normal nonstress level, telling the body that the danger has passed. The behavioral and physical adaptations to short-term stress reverse, and the body returns to its state of rest.

Remember stress physiologist Hans Selye and his mice? Selye concluded that humans under chronic stress become susceptible to disease because they deplete their stress hormone reserves. He believed that if the primal stress response were constantly activated, our bodies would literally run out of protective hormones and we would become defenseless and vulnerable.

Recent research has proved just the opposite to be true. The body *cannot* deplete its stores of the stress hormones. It will keep secreting stress hormones if it is under chronic stress, until a critical threshold is exceeded. Once that happens, the body, as if constantly primed for action, is bathed in waves of these hormones. And if the body cannot return to homeostasis, health begins to break down.

Selye noted that "although we cannot avoid stress as long as we live, we can learn a great deal about how to keep its damaging side effects, 'distress,' to a minimum. For instance, we are just beginning to see that many common diseases are largely due to errors in our adaptive response to stress, rather than to direct damage by germs. In this sense, many nervous and emotional disturbances, high blood pressure, gastric and duodenal ulcers, and certain types of sexual, allergic, cardiovascular, and renal derangements appear to be essentially diseases of adaptation."

Our bodies were never meant to handle long-term stress. We were designed to respond only to immediate, short-term stress. We weren't built to run "hot" all the time. We need the stress response turned down and contained to maintain balance and harmony.

■ Stress and Eating

Stress hormones are invaluable. They make fuel available for the stress response. When the stress response is activated, the adrenaline and cortisol levels rise, together telling the body to release sugar into the bloodstream to give it a surge of energy. The sugar (or glucose) comes from the muscles or liver, where it is stored while waiting to be used, and allows you to perform at your peak. Ask any marathoner! Or a woman running for the last bus after work. It's a key burst of energy, so familiar and necessary.

Adrenaline and cortisol also make fat fuel available. Fat is a high-octane fuel. When you burn 1 gram of carbohydrate fuel, you receive 4 units of energy (calories). When you burn 1 gram of fat, you receive 9 units of energy. Which would you want in your tank? Although both are used under stress, it's fat fuel that enables powerful flight from the man-eating tiger in the jungle.

Adrenaline and cortisol are like a homing device: they zero in on the high-octane fat in the body, alert it to an emergency, and tell it to go into the bloodstream for energy.

Where in the body does the cortisol find the fat? The fat that surrounds your internal organs is the easiest to access, and I call it "Stress Fat." More specifically, we know that Stress Fat has to come from an area close to the portal vein of the liver in the abdomen. This is the case so that the fat fuel can be quickly and efficiently delivered to the liver and converted into fuel to give you the energy for the stress response. The liver is where the fatty acids and triglycerides (fancy names for how fat is stored in fat cells), derived from Stress Fat cells, are converted into fuel. These fat cells, then, are invaluable to the stress response. When adrenaline and cortisol home in on Stress Fat cells, the cells go through a process called "lipolysis," releasing fat from the cells. So it makes sense that the best place to pull fat from for immediate relief is inside your belly.

Stress Fat is different from fat found in other parts of the human body. Normally, it poses no problem. When there is too much of it,

---

Figure 2-4. **How Stress Fat Becomes Toxic Weight**

Stress Fat
⇩
⇩ ⇦ **TOXIC STRESS**
⇩
More Stress Fat Added
⇩
⇩
⇩
TOXIC WEIGHT
⇩
Enlarged Waistline
⇩
Metabolic Syndrome

---

however, it becomes toxic, overwhelming the liver and impairing its daily functions. When this occurs, a variety of metabolic disturbances result, including:

- **High blood sugar**
- **High cholesterol**
- **High blood pressure**
- **High blood coagulability, which predisposes to the formation of blood clots**

These abnormalities lead to serious illnesses, including heart disease and diabetes. The combination of Toxic Weight, heart disease, and diabetes is referred to by medical practitioners as the Metabolic Syndrome, or Syndrome X. Therefore, being apple shaped or carrying the majority of your fat in or around your abdomen is associated with serious illness. The question is, are you at risk for the Metabolic Syndrome?

To determine this, medical scientists have formulated a predictive risk measure called the Waist to Hip Ratio (WHR). To be as precise as possible, measure your waistline at the smallest circumference between the upper part of your hip bone and the lowest part of your rib cage, usually measured on the side of your body. Using a tape, measure that distance. Some women's waistlines are very easy to see and measure while others' are less obvious. The key is to realize that you are at an elevated risk for the Metabolic Syndrome if your waist is 35 inches or greater. For those women whose waists are less than 35 inches, continue to measure your hips by measuring the widest point on your hips. Calculate your WHR by dividing your waist measurement by your hip measurement.

Keep in mind:

■ **WHR less than .8 is optimal**
■ **WHR between .8 and .85 is borderline**
■ **Waist circumference equal to or greater than 35 or WHR greater than .85 indicates you are at risk for Metabolic Syndrome**

Furthermore, stress physiologists, notably Per Björntorp, M.D., have expanded the concept of the Metabolic Syndrome into the "Civilization Syndrome." In this model, Dr. Björntorp combines chronic stress with self-destructive behaviors such as smoking and excess alcohol consumption and has shown that all contribute to the Metabolic Syndrome and are caused by the inability to adapt to the increasing stress of today's society.

After the stress response is over, balance is restored so that the body is prepared for the next stress. Not only do the hormones need to be replenished, but the fuel level needs to be restored. Because you have burned high-octane fat, the body needs to replenish itself. Cortisol sparks your appetite and makes you ravenous (see Figure 2-4).

And what do you crave after stress? Have you ever noticed how it's never a can of tuna we want late at night when we're stressed out? It's always ice cream or a candy bar or cookies. Those foods provide exactly what your body needs: carbohydrates and fat to replenish the calories used up during the stress response—which, in simplest terms, is one of the main ways that activating the stress response on a constant basis can make you fat.

Now that you understand the way our stress response was designed to work—quick burst, immediate response, then cooldown—ask yourself what happens when the stress response runs constantly.

Think of it as the dome light inside your car. If it's late at night and you need to read a map, the car light is helpful. It allows you to check where you are and go on your way. But what happens if you

---

Figure 2-5. **The Fight-or-Flight Response**

Stress and Eating: The Primal Model

Homeostasis
⇩

STRESS
⇩

Stress response activated
⇩

Appetite temporarily shut off
⇩

Cortisol and adrenaline secreted into bloodstream
⇩

**Carbohydrate and fat made available
for fight-or-flight response**
⇩

STRESS RESOLVED
⇩

Stress response subsides
⇩

Adrenaline levels decrease
⇩

Cortisol levels stay elevated to stimulate appetite to refuel
⇩

Poststress refeeding
⇩

Carbohydrate and fat refueled
⇩

Homeostasis restored

---

leave the car light on all night when the car is not running? The car battery dies.

Cortisol, the stress hormone that floods a chronically stressed-out body, is not, however, the enemy it is sometimes portrayed to be. It's a lifesaver, there to keep us moving.

Cortisol is extremely valuable in helping to provide "fight-or-flight" fuel and then, by inducing a poststress appetite, initiate refueling for the next stressful event. It's important to note that before fifty years ago, most daily stressors were physical or required physical responses. Washing clothes by hand required energy. Going to school could involve a two-mile walk in the snow. Putting food on the table might mean a long walk into town to buy provisions, pulling plants from the fields, or milking cows.

We were more in sync with a biological system made for expending fuel and then refueling. Now, because our stressors no longer require physical responses, we are left in a state of perpetual imbalance.

■ Chronic Stress and Fat

Dr. Chrousos and I began our work trying to determine why chronic stress leads to overeating, which then results in the deposition of fat deep inside the abdomen. We chose a rare medical condition called Cushing's Syndrome to help us understand eating and stress. Cushing's Syndrome is a disease caused by prolonged exposure to excessive amounts of cortisol as the result of a tiny tumor that can grow in the brain, in the adrenals, or, not so typically, in other organs such as the lung.

The tumor causes the body to produce high levels of cortisol, which makes the patient ill. Sufferers of Cushing's Syndrome have a unique apple-shaped body, due to the accumulation of large amounts of fat in the belly. Once the tumor is surgically removed, the patient is able to lose the excess intra-abdominal fat and return to health.

Cushing's, we discovered, mimics what would happen if we were walking around with high levels of cortisol for months or years and didn't know it. Chronically elevated levels of cortisol stimulate Stress Fat cells to continually store more fat fuel. This leads to an excessive accumulation of intra-abdominal fat, or Toxic Weight, which, as you recall, is associated with serious medical illnesses, such as diabetes, heart disease, and cancer. This elevation of circulating cortisol also leads to muscle and bone breakdown, as well as suppression of the immune system. Other symptoms are abnormal reproductive function, anxiety, panic attacks, and depression.

Through our studies with Cushing's Syndrome, we came to understand how stress can literally change the shape of your body. As part of our work, we performed computerized tomography (CT) scans of the abdomens of our patients. These pictures gave us an accurate picture of what the fat looks like (see slide 1).

Slide 1 shows the CT scan of a typical obese woman prior to the onset of menopause. This is a special type of CT scan that allows us to highlight the fat as white. This scan was performed while she was lying on her back and "cuts" her at the level of her lower back, or at about lumbar vertebrae 3 to 4, so that you can see her internal organs, bones, and fat. You will notice that most of her fat is the "pinch an inch" variety; it is superficial and falls to her side while she is lying there. It is outside the abdominal muscle wall. There is some inside her abdominal cavity to buffer her organs and keep her warm. If she were now to stand up, you would see that she is a classic pear-shaped woman, with most of her fat on her hips, thighs, and buttocks, and that her waistline fat is mostly abdominal "fluff" on top of the abdominal muscle wall.

Slide 1. **Premenopausal Woman**

Obese Woman—Total Adipose

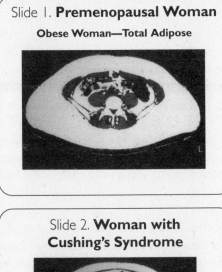

Slide 2 shows a woman with Cushing's Syndrome. Notice how the fat layers are exactly the opposite: she has a tremendous amount of fat inside her abdomen and a very little of the "pinch an inch fluff" characteristic of the classic premenopausal woman! This is because of increased cortisol, which causes fat to be stored deep inside the tummy, creating Toxic Weight.

By the way, this is the same type of picture you would see if you were to perform a CT scan of an overweight baby-boomer male. Men are born with

Slide 2. **Woman with Cushing's Syndrome**

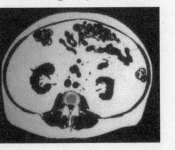

more fat cells inside the abdomen and preferentially store fat there. As they accumulate fat through poor lifestyle habits as well as increasing stress and declining testosterone levels, the majority of the fat goes deep inside the abdomen as Toxic Weight. This is one reason why so many men are vulnerable to heart disease, high blood pressure, and diabetes as they pile on weight. Menopausal women, as we shall see, can begin to look like their apple-shaped male counterparts as they age. Declining estrogen levels, increasing stress, and poor lifestyle habits stimulate fat accumulation inside the abdomen for them as well.

Interestingly, not all people with Cushing's Syndrome become fat. How can that be? Some individuals never knew they had the disease but noted that their weight was up a bit and decided to fight the fat through vigorous exercise and careful eating. Is it possible to counteract the powerful forces of extremely high levels of cortisol?

I stumbled upon the answer when I met an extraordinary young woman who was about twenty years old and was admitted to the hospital with fulminant Cushing's Syndrome caused by tumors in both of her adrenal glands. She didn't even know she had the problem until she fractured a bone while running and the physician looking at her X rays noted that her bones appeared brittle, a classic result of prolonged exposure to high levels of stress hormones. I recall that whenever I tried to find her to perform a medical history and physical, she was never in her room. The nurses told me that if I wanted to locate her, I should stand at the top of the tenth-floor stairwell and shout her name. Baffled but intrigued, I did so. Sure enough, there she was, running up and down the stairs. Fascinated, I asked her why she was doing this. Smiling and energetic, she replied that it was the only thing that made her feel better. As it turned out, she was an athlete and used her physical activity as well as controlled eating habits to literally neutralize her high levels of stress hormones. How? The beta-endorphin dopamine and serotonin secreted as a result of vigorous physical activity helped calm down the stress response that was running rampant in her body. Exercise also diminished her feelings of anxiety and depression. "Better living through your own chemicals," she would often say jokingly.

But most interesting was the fact that although she did gain some weight, she controlled that weight gain with her athleticism and dietary habits. Her CT scan (see slide 3) looks like that of an average, athletic young woman with minimal superficial fat and without excessive intra-

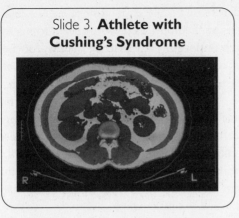

Slide 3. **Athlete with Cushing's Syndrome**

abdominal fat. Yet the extremely high levels of cortisol coursing through her body were as treacherous as a walk through a minefield.

Lesson learned? There is no question that stress can make you fat, especially deep inside the abdomen. There is also no question that a healthy lifestyle can counteract this effect.

In the laboratory, I worked with fat cells that I obtained during surgery on Cushing's patients and compared them to the fat cells of normal volunteers (see slide 4 of fat cells). As you can see, fat cells look like big soap bubbles. Each fat cell comes equipped with two doors, an "entrance" and an "exit." Each one has a separate key. The entrance door allows fat to be stored and is controlled by an enzyme called lipoprotein lipase (LPL). The exit door allows fat to leave, and its gatekeeper is an enzyme called hormone-sensitive lipase (HSL). Fat cell synthesis is the process of filling up the cell with fat fuel. Consuming too many calories stimulates the body to store fat. Fat cell lipolysis is the term for the process of a fat cell's release of its fuel into the bloodstream. Physical activity, such as walking, promotes lipolysis. When you lose weight, your fat cells empty out and collapse. But they don't go away, they wait to be filled again. In collapsed fat cell

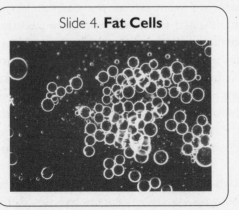

Slide 4. **Fat Cells**

mode, you can fit into your Calvin Klein jeans. In filled-up mode, you can't.

A variety of chemicals and hormones in your body control fat storage and release. Using molecular biology techniques, we found that fat cells have special stress hormone receptors for cortisol. There seem to be more of these on the intra-abdominal fat cells than on fat cells in other parts of the body. This would seem to make sense, since this fat depot is so important in providing the fuel for the stress response. Those cells should be very responsive to cortisol when it orders them either to release their precious fuel into the bloodstream for the "fight-or-flight" response or to refuel and store fat. However, fat cells exposed to high levels of cortisol for too long go through changes. Under chronic stress, insulin, a fat storage hormone, rises and, in combination with high levels of cortisol, promotes fat storage and inhibits fat release. That's one of the main reasons that during chronic stress fat is stored deep inside the abdomen.

Research tells us that prolonged exposure of Stress Fat to high levels of cortisol makes Stress Fat cells more sensitive and responsive to stress hormones, resulting in a greater tendency to build Toxic Weight. Moreover, this process may actually begin to occur as early as *in utero*. Animals that have been administered the equivalent of cortisol during their pregnancy deliver babies that are very hypersensitive to stress and prone to abnormal behaviors as they mature.

Research also now shows that chronically stressed people can't think clearly. They have a decreased immune system response—for example, increased susceptibility to the common cold. People undergoing interpersonal stresses at home or work show a similar immune suppression. Studies also show that men who are under severe stress experience a higher rate of heart attacks. Furthermore, stressed-out people sleep poorly and show signs of depression and anxiety. In a study of Volvo employees, Swedish researchers found that the female employees had high stress levels. They measured the women's blood pressure and levels of adrenaline and found that both remained elevated long after the end of the workday while the men's decreased soon after they left work. This indicates that women's stress hormones remain elevated as they anticipate further and continuing stresses resulting from family obligations or other concerns after they leave work. The Toxic Stress of continually trying to live up to work and family obligations and expectations often leaves women feeling chronically burnt out and guilty whether they fail or succeed in achieving their goals.

When the body is exposed to high levels of stress hormones on a chronic basis, every physiological system is affected (see Box 2-1).

Box 2-1. **Effects of Long-term Exposure to High Levels of Cortisol**

- Impaired immune response: increased risk of infection, inflammatory and autoimmune conditions, and possibly cancer
- Changes in body composition: decreased muscle mass and increased fat deposition inside the abdomen, decreased bone density (increased risk of osteoporosis)
- Mental health problems: suppression of reward systems, increased risk of depression, anxiety, shifting moods of anger and frustration
- Memory and learning impairment
- Sleep impairment
- Increased risk of heart attack
- Reproductive dysfunctions: irregular menstrual cycles, decreased fertility, premenstrual syndrome (PMS), increased risk of postpartum depression, increased discomfort in the perimenopause
- Altered eating patterns: most frequently, overeating and weight gain; less frequently, undereating and weight loss followed by weight gain

---

■ Perimenopausal Weight Gain

A woman sits at her desk while her boss chastises her for missing an important deadline. She tells the boss she had to take her daughter to the doctor for a strep test that morning. "You'll never get anywhere in this organization until you get your priorities straight," the boss says chillingly.

What would you do?

Studies done by Redford Williams and his colleagues at Duke University have shown that most women would sit there and take it. Obsessing about the hurt and humiliation, they then experience a growing appetite. They begin to yearn for food and are likely to begin snacking during the afternoon, visiting the vending machines or the company kitchen, hunting for goodies.

What's going on here, and what are the options? To answer this, let's look at the stress and eating model as we enter the twenty-first century. We have turned the "fight-or-flight" response into the "stew-and-chew" response (see Figure 2-6).

If the woman whose boss chastised her about missing work had

Figure 2-6. **The Stew-and-Chew Response**

Stress and Eating: The Twenty-first-Century Model

Homeostasis
⇩
STRESS
⇩
Stress response activated
⇩
Appetite temporarily shut off
⇩
Adrenaline and cortisol secreted into bloodstream
⇩
Make carbohydrates and fat available
for fight-or-flight response
⇩
STRESS UNRESOLVED
⇩
TOXIC STRESS
⇩
Stress response continues
⇩
Adrenaline levels stay elevated, keeping blood pressure high
⇩
Cortisol levels stay elevated and stimulate appetite
⇩
STRESS EATING
⇩
Carbohydrates and/or fat eaten excessively
⇩
TOXIC WEIGHT GAIN
⇩
Homeostasis not restored

been able to fulfill her genetic destiny, she would have gotten up and fought back. She would have done something physical! After all, calories were pouring through her blood vessels, preparing her for action.

When the Alarm Hormone is released by the stress of a confrontation, the hormonal cascade begins as it was designed. But no physical response follows. The body, however, does not signal the brain that a physical response did not take place. As far as the brain is concerned, the stress-response cycle must be completed. And the stress response always results in a cortisol-induced appetite to replenish the fuel that was supposedly burned, whether or not a physical response has taken place. This relentless refueling appetite continues until the stress is resolved. However, if the stress remains unresolved, the chronically elevated levels of stress hormones not only stimulate appetite but also encourage Stress Fat cells deep inside the abdomen to store more fat. Excess accumulations of this intra-abdominal fat are Toxic Weight.

Most women over the age of forty, including athletes and other women who try to stay in good shape, notice they are gaining weight, primarily around the abdomen. The fat is deposited at the waist, and suddenly belts are a thing of the past and jeans don't zip anymore.

Women over forty are especially vulnerable to Toxic Weight gain. This is because of the influence of chronic Toxic Stress in their lives, as well as the metabolic and hormonal changes they undergo during perimenopause.

In case you think that only humans have a problem with stewing and chewing, as far back as twenty years ago researchers discovered that animals also demonstrate a chewing response when under stress. Dr. James Morley and Dr. Allen Levine, in their famous tail-pinch experiments, found that rats under experimental stress increased their consumption of food, even when already satisfied from a prior feeding—and furthermore, they preferred carbohydrates and fat in these stress-induced meals.

■ Metabolism

One of the biggest reasons women over forty gain weight is that they become metabolically cooler. We simply don't burn calories as efficiently as we did a decade ago. Even women who exercise regularly notice the extra weight accumulating around their waists. The metabolic drop has actually been occurring for years, ever since the age of twenty, when growth hormone settled down. The basal metabolic rate drops by approximately 5 percent per decade of life. When a woman hits forty, she is entering her third 5 percent decrease. In addition, postmenopausal women are at higher risk for hypothyroidism than younger women, which also has an impact on their metabolism, making it more of a challenge to lose weight during this period of life.

At the same time, we experience one of the greatest drops of muscle mass in our lives. As a woman enters her forties, she is more sedentary. Chasing after the kids or carrying them around is less common. And with a woman's busy schedule, it seems there is simply no time to exercise. But the price she pays for this sedentary lifestyle is a loss of more than seven pounds of muscle every ten years. And since muscle mass is her calorie-burning furnace this means she has lost the ability to burn approximately 400 calories per day.

Dieting can also contribute to loss of muscle mass. When the body goes into "starvation" mode, it uses valuable muscle mass to provide energy since calories are not coming from any other source.

Weight gain in menopause was not studied extensively by researchers until recently. Before this, women naively thought they could maintain the same body composition they had in their twenties and thirties—and, of course, rely on crash diets for a quick fix.

Researchers at the University of Pittsburgh studied weight changes in more than five hundred middle-aged women. Not surprisingly, the greatest weight gains were among the women who were the most sedentary. This pointed the finger not at menopause but at lack of physical activity.

When a woman passes through menopause, her energy requirement is about 15 percent less than it was when she was in her twenties. So if we eat the same way at age fifty-five that we did at age twenty-five, we are sure to gain weight.

■ Cortisol and Menopause Hormones

What happens to a woman's weight during perimenopause, that time between having regular periods and having no periods at all? It can

be a roller-coaster ride, thanks to declining estrogen and progesterone levels. Estrogen tends to hold fluid in the body while progesterone has a mild diuretic effect. In the normal menstrual cycle,
bloating is most severe around the thirteenth or fourteenth day of the
cycle, when estrogen is at its peak. As progesterone slowly rises, there
is some water loss but bloating continues. A week before menstruation, estrogen peaks again and progesterone starts to decline. The result is feeling bloated and noticing that the skirt that fit just fine in the
morning grips like a tourniquet by afternoon.

Why are women at greater risk of developing Toxic Weight? In
premenopausal women, estrogen is a powerful activator of fat storage
in the hips, thighs, and buttocks. The purpose of this fat deposition in
the lower region of the body is primarily the storage of fat for breast-
feeding. Things change during the perimenopause. Estrogen levels become more erratic, waxing and waning, and the storage site of fat
shifts to the abdomen. The fat itself is the soft, fluffy "pinch an inch"
fat outside the abdominal muscle, what I refer to as the "menopot"
(see Figure 2-7). As long as a woman remains physically fit, it does not
seem to be associated with any significant or life-threatening disease.
Even athletes find it difficult not to gain some weight during the perimenopause. This appears to be a fairly normal and natural occurrence
in women over forty-five. If, however, a perimenopausal woman is

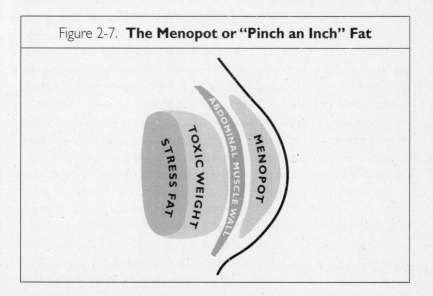

Figure 2-7. **The Menopot or "Pinch an Inch" Fat**

afflicted by Toxic Stress, fat will also be deposited deep inside the belly, forming Toxic Weight. Therefore, the weight gain of the peri-menopause can be distributed into two abdominal depots: the subcu-taneous fluff of the menopot and the deep, internal Toxic Weight.

Declining estrogen and progesterone are not the only hormones of importance during perimenopause. The ovaries secrete testos-terone as well. As levels of the other sex hormones decline, testos-terone levels become more predominant relative to the decreasing estrogen and progesterone. Testosterone is a potent stimulant of intra-abdominal fat deposition, resulting in the potential for a buildup of excess Stress Fat, or Toxic Weight.

But it isn't just lowered metabolism and decreased hormonal lev-els that cause women's weight gain in their forties. The stress hor-mone cortisol also plays an important role. We know that Toxic Stress produces a constant flood of cortisol. We also know that ab-normally prolonged cortisol secretion stimulates the hormone in-sulin. During chronic stress, insulin, a powerful fat storage hormone, short-circuits the release of fat stimulated by adrenaline and cortisol and encourages fat storage, specifically inside the abdomen. Current studies have shown that women in menopause have higher circulat-ing levels of insulin and thus a greater propensity to store fat. Also, women at this age do not process carbohydrates (sugar, glucose) as well as younger women, which further increases their insulin levels. In addition, the high levels of cortisol, stimulated by chronic stress, facilitate insulin's fat storage in Stress Fat cells.

Insulin isn't the only culprit. A woman accumulates fat after forty because other fat regulators, including growth hormone and leptin, are also declining. For most of their lives, women have been told that estrogen and progesterone are the key hormones controlling every-thing from body shape to mood swings. But there's more. As it turns out, stress hormones play a pivotal role in hormonal changes throughout a woman's life (see Figure 2-8). Stress hormones and estrogen are closely associated, like best friends. Actually, stress hor-mones determine how well we cope with all of the hormonal mile-stones in our lives. When we begin to menstruate, stress hormones can affect our mood, the severity of PMS and cramping, as well as our appetite during menstruation. During pregnancy, our stress hor-mone levels may predispose us to postpartum depression.

During the perimenopause, as estrogen begins to decline signifi-

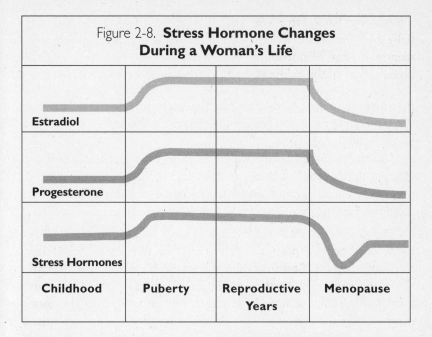

Figure 2-8. **Stress Hormone Changes During a Woman's Life**

Estradiol			
Progesterone			
Stress Hormones			
Childhood	Puberty	Reproductive Years	Menopause

cantly, the stress hormones decrease as well. Studies measuring morning cortisol indicate that levels of this hormone are decreased by 40 to 50 percent. The activation system is dimmed. How long does this last? Researchers have shown that it may last up to one year, after which time the body seems to adapt to the lower levels of estrogen. During this period of time, when the stress-response hormones are temporarily operating at a significantly lower level, women are vulnerable to the consequences of less hormone availability. This may account for the striking lack of energy and mood disturbances so many women feel in the perimenopause, regardless of their level of fitness.

The good news is that the stress hormone levels do become reestablished, but at a lower level compared to the premenopausal period. This somewhat lowered activation level is one of the reasons why, as we age, we may feel slightly less energetic than we once did.

■ Syndrome W

By now you should appreciate the fact that women after the age of forty gain weight around their waistlines because of:

- ■ **Aging metabolism**
- ■ **Lifestyle choices**
- ■ **Chronic Toxic Stress**
- ■ **Hormone changes**

After the age of forty, the weight gain issue changes. The question is no longer how fat one is. Now, in the perimenopause, it's where the fat is located.

As we have seen, as a woman ages, it's the excess fat, the Toxic Weight that settles inside her abdomen, that for the first time in her life, places her at great risk for early disease and death. Recall that medical practitioners have referred to the combination of Toxic Weight, heart disease, and diabetes as the Metabolic Syndrome. Until recently, no distinction was made between how men and women succumb to the ills of the Metabolic Syndrome. Perimenopausal women are, in fact, unique. Their Toxic Weight and its consequences during this time of life can be referred to as "Syndrome W":

- ■ **Women (hormones)**
- ■ **Worry (Toxic Stress)**
- ■ **Weight (gain)**
- ■ **Waist (Toxic Weight)**

It's an easy way to connect the effect your mind (worry and chronic stress) has on your perimenopausal body (weight gain in the waist). Syndrome W reminds women to be acutely aware of the role that chronic Toxic Stress plays, not only in weight gain but in potentially shortening their lives. The "worry" component of Syndrome W and its potent effect on Toxic Weight gain have never before been empha- sized. Now we know that stress puts on fat, primarily as Toxic Weight.

Thinking about Syndrome W can encourage you to go back and reassess the factors in your life that you can change to minimize any accumulation of Toxic Weight. Learning how to become more Stress- Resilient in your daily life is the key to starting that journey.

Here are a few inescapable conclusions for the average woman:

- ■ **The average weight gain during the perimenopausal period (spanning five to ten years) can be 2 to 3 pounds per
  year or more. Though there are conflicting research data**

as to why this occurs, we are beginning to understand the connections among age, hormonal status, and lifestyle. Women who exercise regularly have minimal weight gain throughout menopause.

■ This weight gain is accompanied by an increase in the amount of total body fat, especially in the upper body and primarily in the abdominal region. This redistribution of fat from the thighs to the abdomen results in an increase in the waist-to-hip ratio, or a transformation of the body from pear- to apple-shaped.

■ Muscle mass declines. If you do not use it, you lose it. Women lose more than seven pounds of solid muscle mass per decade of adult life if they do not do enough physical activity.

So while hormones, lifestyle choices, and aging all play a part, Toxic Stress can *trigger* additional Toxic Weight gain in a woman over forty. And that fat heads straight to the waist—which is why developing a more Stress-Resilient personality is important for everyone, but absolutely critical for women over the age of forty.

The question is not one of vanity; it's one of saving your life.

3 The Itch You Can't Scratch—Pinpoint Your Stress-Eating Profile

During the last seven years of working with stress eaters, many of my patients have told me I was their "last hope." I suppose that's my greatest strength as a doctor: offering people hope.

As the issue of weight and stress gained in popularity, I was sought out by reporters for my observations in numerous magazine articles on the subject. After each article appeared, my phone would ring off the hook. My mailbox became stuffed with urgent letters. It was clear there was a real need for information.

Whenever a new patient walked into my office, she was convinced there was something wrong with her. At the age of forty, why, she wondered, couldn't she lose weight?

While each patient is unique, all share a similar sense of hopelessness. The first thing I ask of each of them is the most crucial: a commitment to self-care. I know they are all veterans of the diet wars. They know all the dietspeak: "I cheated . . . I'll start again in the morning . . ." They are so familiar with the false promises of temporary fixes that they have no idea how to begin a long-term plan—how to save the second half of their lives.

But now they know. And I want to share with you some of their thoughts and insights as we examine stress eating and determine your stress profile. Every woman's stress triggers are different, but many women share the same stress profile.

I invited a dozen of my patients to gather one evening after work to discuss the topic "Women, Weight, and Stress." All of them had been my patients for at least three or four months, some for as long as five years, and they were in varying stages of their self-care journey. One of the first questions I threw out sparked the beginning of a lively session that lasted for hours. The discussion began with shared recollections of shopping in the Chubbette Department, evolved into a confessional of painful memories (such as always being told, "You have such a pretty face"), and ended with tearful embraces.

The first provocative question: In what ways do men and women react differently to stress?

"Men yell," Karen said. "Men scream."

"Women internalize," offered Marcia.

"Or shop," said Eileen with a laugh.

"Men push back. Women swallow it," came another voice.

"Women *eat*!" yelled Barbara.

I then asked them what they said to themselves when they did give in to stress eating.

"I earned it."

"I deserve it."

"I'll just have a little taste. Oh well, I guess I just might as well finish it."

"I actually believe I can eat through my stress."

I asked them what they ate when they had the blues.

"Chocolate!" several women replied in unison. (Bread and other carbohydrates such as pasta were also mentioned.)

Do they ever feel satisfied?

There was dead silence.

"No. When I start to eat, I don't stop."

"Never."

"There seems to be no cue to stop."

"I never have the feeling that I'm full."

"I don't stop until I'm nauseous."

It was Barbara who best described the feeling of emptiness, the void that can never be filled, the insatiable aspect of stress hunger: "It's like you can't scratch that itch."

As all the evidence pointed to stress as the culprit, I explained how the feeling of emptiness is related to the stress hormones. No matter how much these women ate, the feelings of fulfillment, reward, and satiety were missing. They had broken "feedometers" that started at "starved" and then zoomed ahead to "stuffed," without ever braking at "full."

Often intent on anesthetizing pain, many of the women confessed to eating until they felt physically sick. They eat fast. They do not taste or savor their food. They gulp and overconsume. They circumvent the relay system that delicately attaches to the top of the brain and says "I'm full."

The Alarm Hormone and cortisol are out of balance in these women. There's a neurochemical disconnection. They have no braking system, and that sets up a vicious stress-eating cycle (see Figure 3-1).

After grasping this concept, these women finally realize there are no instant results. They know they have never before been given a chance to succeed. They know that food can no longer be an anesthetic. They understand the stress response and how it works. They know eating and weight loss are not just about willpower but the fact that a healthy body resonates from a healthy mind. If the brain never registers the reward of being "full," it will tell the stomach to continue eating.

As we went around the table and heard the women's stories, I was moved by how secure they felt about sharing their experiences. I

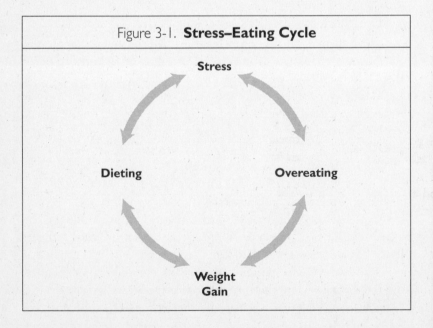

Figure 3-1. **Stress–Eating Cycle**

Stress

Overeating

Weight
Gain

Dieting

was also proud that they no longer measured their success or failure by the scale but instead by their newly found inner power to fight for their survival. They have all learned to trade in the unsatisfying "rewards" of food for other, real rewards that are truly fulfilling. Teaching them to stop substituting rich food for a rich life is part of my job as their "nutrishrink." I also help them make a commitment to care for themselves.

"If you're putting yourself last on the list," one of the women observed, "it's much harder to handle stress."

Exercise has become nonnegotiable for all of them. Mindless foraging is a thing of the past. "Understanding that this is not a diet," said Barbara. "It is a way of life."

Most important, they have all learned the secrets of recovering after a lapse. "The one thing that has helped me," said Karen, "is knowing I have a day or two to regroup and not to see this as a failure or to completely throw in the towel and say all those negative things I would say: I cheated; I failed."

Once these women made the connection between food and stress, they were able to understand that each of them has a different "stress profile" that determines their eating patterns.

Biologically speaking, the stress response, which affects our eating and sleeping habits, is determined by the cluster of stress hormones, from the Alarm Hormone in the brain to cortisol and adrenaline in the bloodstream. And the stress hormones control the reward system (which you'll remember from Chapter 2 is the biological sense of feeling satiated and rewarded). So it makes sense that the Alarm Hormone, which acts as an appetite suppressant, and cortisol, which acts as an appetite stimulant, have major effects on eating. But how can these two stress hormones, with their antithetical actions on appetite, coexist?

Each woman's response to food in the face of stress is different. After a particularly hectic day, some women can't choke down a sandwich while others are ravenous.

A doctor once told me, "Rosie, you're overweight." I said, "I know." He said, "Here's what you have to do. Instead of eating Oreos, eat carrots." It's so simplistic to think that being fat is only about the food you put into your mouth, because it's really about control and feeling safe. I was enraged. I said to the doctor, "It's so insulting of you to think that you just cured obesity in America. Thank you. You're a genius. Fat people had no idea that carrots are better for you than Ring-Dings. Who knew?"

—Rosie O'Donnell interview, *Marie Claire*, June 1999

Gaining control and feeling safe: that is exactly how you can learn to deal with stress in your life. That's why Rosie's doctor's advice was so simplistic. Being fat is rarely about carrots versus Oreos. It's about what you do with your mouth when life seems tough.

Let me ask you a question: After a particularly stressful day, which of the following are you likely to do?

1. **Take a bath, hop into bed, and bury yourself in a good book.**
2. **Wander mindlessly into the kitchen in a trance, open the freezer, take out a gallon of jamocha chip nut fudge ice cream, and begin a feeding frenzy because you "deserve it."**
3. **Forget the ice cream. Forget food at all. Skip dinner, pace nervously around the house, go to bed anxious, and barely sleep.**

These are examples of typical behavior patterns of what I see as the three eating responses to stress. I refer to them as the three "Stress-Eating Profiles."

1. **Stress-Resilient (healthy eaters)**
2. **Stress Overeaters**
3. **Stress Undereaters**

Here's how these behavior patterns work.

First, the brain releases a message to a small vascular system that connects the hypothalamus to the pituitary gland. This message is sent from the Alarm Hormone. Within seconds, it triggers the pituitary gland to secrete ACTH (adrenocortotropic hormone, or corticotropin). The ACTH shoots to the adrenal gland, and within minutes glucocorticoids are released. Simultaneously, the Alarm Hormone stimulates nerves in the brain stem that communicate with the spinal cord and finally tell the adrenal glands to secrete adrenaline.

If you're *Stress-Resilient*, when you're under stress you cope well, and a normal amount of Alarm Hormone is secreted and a normal secretion of adrenaline and cortisol follows. Your body remains in balance. There is no excess of either hormone. Cortisol does not linger in your system.

Stress Overeaters are often born with a smaller than normal or inadequate amount of the Alarm Hormone. It can send only a faint message to the adrenal glands. Because of this, the stress response in some people, Dr. Chrousos has found, doesn't work right. Indeed, if you are a Stress Overeater, the lack of appropriate level of the Alarm Hormone makes you feel as though you are not complete or full. It's like a dull, constant ache.

The initial "spark" from the Alarm Hormone that occurs when you are under stress is not strong enough to initiate a healthy cascade of hormones into your blood. It "undershoots" the stress response. Because your body needs the stress hormones to react properly to stress, close to normal amounts of cortisol will be secreted. The secretion of the less than adequate amount of Alarm Hormone, combined with the normal secretion of cortisol, which is slower to be released and cleared from the bloodstream, leads to appetite stimulation.

Stress Overeaters also respond to chronic stress by inappropriate eating because their "reward" system is not operating correctly and because there's not enough Alarm Hormone to neutralize the appetite stimulation caused by cortisol. They are likely to binge-eat to quench their need for reward and fulfillment, but of course they never feel adequately satisfied.

If you are a *Stress Undereater,* you were born with higher than normal levels of Alarm Hormone. When you're under stress, a message is sent to the adrenals to secrete both adrenaline and cortisol continually. Since the Alarm Hormone is one of the most potent appetite suppressants we know of, your biological instinct is to reject food.

In each stress-eating profile, stress triggers different adaptive responses based on genetics and environment. These characteristics include what happens with your Alarm Hormone and cortisol and how, under the chronic stress of daily life, these hormones affect your

1. **Eating patterns (healthy versus unhealthy)**
2. **Sleeping patterns**
3. **Body composition, including fat, muscle, and the presence or absence of Toxic Weight**

4. **Body Mass Index (BMI)**
5. **Fitness level**
6. **Psychological state**
7. **Reward-seeking behavior**
8. **Ability to neutralize your stress eating**

For each of the three stress-eating profiles I have prepared a clinical evaluation with a list of basic helpful tips to guide each profile as she navigates through the day. Following those are prescriptions in which you will notice references to the "CortiZone." Recall from Chapter 2 that cortisol and the stress hormones in general follow a daily biorhythm in which their levels peak in the morning and are lowest during sleep. Starting at approximately 3 to 4 P.M. and continuing until midnight, they decrease, making it more difficult for you to pay attention and be mindful of your self-care. I refer to this period as the "CortiZone." It is a time during which all stress profiles are vulnerable to abnormal stress-induced eating behaviors. Study the stress profile prescriptions in Chapter 10 and their relation to the CortiZone, as we will be revisiting the CortiZone in more detail throughout each template in Part II.

In the program found in Part II, specific prescriptions will be provided guiding each stress profile as she copes with daily stresses.

Keep in mind as you review the stress profiles that most people move among the three profiles at various points in their lives, but everyone tends eventually to return to his or her original inclination (see Figure 3-2).

The stress profiles of some women will overlap, depending on their life experiences. And some women's stress profiles will vary de-

---

Figure 3-2. **Revisiting the Stress Profiles Throughout Life**

(Goal)

Stress-Resilient

⇩ ⇧   ⇩ ⇧

⇩ ⇧   ⇩ ⇧

Stress Overeater ⇦⇦⇨⇨ **Stress Undereater**

pending on their menstrual cycle. Women who are Stress-Resilient may sometimes undergo stress cravings during PMS. That is normal and to be expected. The goal is to be Stress-Resilient at least 50 percent of the time, which is the first profile.

■ I. Stress-Resilient

(See Box 3-1 for clinical evaluation.)

Those who fall under the *Stress-Resilient* profile are the master "regroupers": whatever life dishes out, they make do, adapt, and cope without self-destruction. Through experience, they have achieved the ability to control their stress response without overeating or deprivation. Their body's hormonal system remains in balance. Their appetite is in check. Food is neither a reward nor a punishment.

Why? When stress hits, the brain shoots a normal amount of the Alarm Hormone into their system, releasing a normal amount of

Box 3-1. **Clinical Evaluation: Stress-Resilient**	
Alarm Hormone	Healthy range
Cortisol	Healthy range
Eating behavior	Healthy and appropriate
Sleeping pattern	Normal
Body composition after forty	Healthy weight, muscle mass, and fat mass; no Toxic Weight; mild to moderate menopot
Body Mass Index	Variable, but no extremes
Physical fitness level	Fit for age
Mental and emotional state	Normal energy level; ability to regroup under life stresses; realistic attitude toward and expectations about life; excellent at coping and adapting; emotionally balanced, not depressed
Reward system	Intact; does not seek satisfaction and fulfillment from food to help cope with stress

adrenaline and cortisol from the adrenal glands in the abdomen. Once the stress is over, the hormones return to their prestress levels and the system returns to balance.

Even in the case of life-threatening stress, they deal with and process the event appropriately. A Stress-Resilient person tries not to harbor Toxic Stress or chronically elevated cortisol. Instead, her priority is to rise to the occasion and cope with whatever challenge is at hand, whether a lost key or the loss of something more devastating such as a loved one. The goal is to return to homeostasis as soon as possible. Neither the hunger response nor the starvation response remains chronically activated. Eating is a moot point.

I don't want to confuse you, but Stress-Resilient people may still become overweight. They may be genetically obese and just not well informed when it comes to eating and exercise. They may be 20 or 30 pounds overweight. But they handle stress fairly well. They are often just mindless about their bodies. They need to be "jump-started" before their lack of physical fitness gets them into perimenopausal trouble. When these women come into my office, I watch what happens as I walk them through the initial stages of the program. They are usually the quickest to catch on to what they have been doing wrong, and they adjust rapidly.

The majority of these women hear my message, make the appropriate changes, and weather the transition, making only a minimal amount of emotional investment in the process.

These "adapters" usually have a high energy level and may be more physically active than others. They move around and neutralize daily stresses as they occur. They don't turn fitness into a second career. They tend not to obsess about self-care. They are not in danger of developing Toxic Stress or Toxic Weight. They tend to have fewer health and emotional problems and enjoy greater longevity.

The current population of centenarians is a wonderful example of an ever-expanding group of Stress-Resilient people who have weathered life's storms and triumphs for a hundred years or more. If you have aspirations of doing the same, now is the time to start!

One important distinction: even though Stress-Resilient women do not develop Toxic Weight, it is normal for them to develop "fluff," or subcutaneous fat, around the waist, to the tune of one to ten pounds. As you recall from Chapter 2, I refer to this as the "menopot."

The Stress-Resilient woman has a Body Mass Index (BMI, or

weight in relation to height) that is not extremely small or large but within ±5 points of the average of 25. Researchers would argue that they should be as close to 25 as possible, but I'm convinced that it is possible to be physically fit and Stress-Resilient, and in general do quite well, at other BMIs. We will discuss this further in the Nutrition Template, Chapter 6. The fit, Stress-Resilient person is not obese or overly thin but of generally average weight for her age, gender, and height.

$$\text{Body Mass Index} = \frac{\text{weight in kilograms}}{\text{height m}^2}$$

Clinical researchers use the following guidelines regarding BMI: 26–30 indicates moderately overweight; 31–39 indicates obese; and 40 or greater indicates seriously obese.

As a group, Stress-Resilient people are extremely in touch with their surroundings and reactions to life events. They see the majority of life's stressors as annoying but livable, not chronic, Toxic Stress. This personality trait can be learned.

Case Study—Eileen, Age Fifty

"I don't see stress as all bad," says Eileen. "There's positive stress, which is very invigorating, such as when I'm on deadline for some exciting project. I can work for hours and not think about food at all. Then there's negative stress, which usually has some emotional problem associated with it: arguments with the kids, conflicts in general. I remember after one argument I had with my son when he was a teenager, I was so upset I had my hand in a cereal box shoveling out some icky sugar-coated flakes I didn't even like. Luckily, we don't fight very often. Perhaps the difference is in my perceived 'control' of the stress. I used to turn to food as a comfort, even though I realized it was only a temporary reprieve from dealing with the problem. I have learned to deal with my problems in a non-self-destructive way. It's about finding constructive (rather than destructive) strategies for dealing with the big and little zingers that life throws your way."

■ 2. Stress Overeaters

(See Box 3-2 for clinical evaluation.)

The majority of over-forty women I see in my practice are *Stress Overeaters*, and the Toxic Stress they harbor signals their bodies to store fat for the physical fight-or-flight response that never takes place. Instead, most often they respond to stress by "stewing and chewing" and are at risk of obesity as well as the accumulation of Toxic Weight. This is why stress eating is the itch you can't scratch.

Stress Overeaters often eat until they feel sick, as they fruitlessly seek reward and anesthesia from the pain of dealing with the chronic stresses in their daily life. This is not a result of real hunger; it's stress-driven appetite caused by chronically inadequate levels of the Alarm Hormone combined with normal cortisol levels. These women's appetites become insatiable because nothing satisfies their constant need for anesthesia. Many also harbor one or more obesity genes, which affects their ability to feel true fullness and satisfaction from eating.

Stress Overeaters were born with lower than normal levels of the Alarm Hormone. They usually have enough for the baseline, lower-stress events of life. But when challenged by short-term stress, they tend to undershoot the stress response, putting out a higher than normal but still less than adequate amount of the Alarm Hormone to cope with it. Dr. Chrousos likes to refer to their stress response as "dim," as if someone had turned down their lights at birth. These women need activation.

When the Alarm Hormone secretion is elevated but still inadequate, what happens to the secretion of cortisol? Is it also less than normal in response to stress? The answer is no. The body has unique sensors to detect inadequate levels of cortisol. Sensing this, it has backup mechanisms that kick in and bring the cortisol level up to par, with normal rises during stress coping. As a result, the level of Alarm Hormone is lower than the level of cortisol, causing an imbalance. Because cortisol stimulates appetite, this imbalance leads to overfeeding.

Unless they can neutralize their stress response, Stress Overeaters will always be out of balance hormonally. When they do not understand the facts behind their condition, Stress Overeaters seek ways to get more activated, more energetic, more alive. Unfortunately, that activation often manifests itself in self-destructive ways, through

Box 3-2. **Clinical Evaluation: Stress Overeaters**

Alarm Hormone	Less than normal
Cortisol	Normal
Eating behavior	Excessive intake of carbohydrate and fat, stimulated by low levels of Alarm Hormone combined with normal levels of cortisol
Sleeping pattern	Normal to excessive sleep; often feels tired upon awakening
Body composition after forty	Overweight or obese, variable fat and lean body mass; moderate to large menopot; Toxic Weight present
Body Mass Index	Above average to very high
Physical fitness level	Unfit
Mental and emotional state	Lower than normal energy; fatigued, atypical depression or functional depression usually present; difficulty regrouping after stress; unrealistic expectations; perfectionism
Reward system	Inadequate; constantly seeking satisfaction and stress relief from food

risk-taking behaviors that include smoking or drinking copious amounts of coffee or alcohol. Stress Overeaters discover that food activates them as well. After years of harboring this chronically disturbed stress system, with lower than normal levels of Alarm Hormone combined with normal levels of cortisol, their bodies are primed for obesity, including Toxic Weight deposition as a result of chronic overeating.

Since Stress Overeaters have dimmed responses to stress in general, they wake up more tired, feel less energetic in the morning, tend to oversleep, and often feel fatigued by midafternoon, forcing them to seek activation, most often by consuming fatty, high-sugar foods or caffeine. They also tend not to be particularly physical or athletic, finding that exercise is hard to initiate and maintain.

Stress Overeaters' body composition is variable, since many have a history of dieting, resulting in major shifts in fat and muscle mass. Most are overweight or obese and thus have an elevated BMI. Most have adequate bone mass since their overweight creates built-in "weight lifting," stimulating their bones to remain strong.

Psychologically, many Stress Overeaters are depressed. This depression may not be great enough to significantly interfere with daily activities and is referred to as subclinical depression. When depression becomes great enough to affect functioning, Stress Overeaters are often diagnosed with atypical depression, which is characterized by lethargy and low energy and is usually associated with little physical activity and often significant weight gain. These women are frequently treated with antidepressants and psychotherapy. In women who suffer from either atypical or subclinical depression, their genetic and environmental backgrounds make them more vulnerable to stress-related eating behaviors because of the sense of despair that accompanies depression. Stress Overeaters' reward systems, like their Alarm Hormone responses, do not function adequately. There is that itch, and you can never scratch it. Chronic caregivers are among the highest group of Stress Overeaters.

Case Study—Gena, Age Forty

"I'm constantly wrestling with the balance of caregiving for others and myself," relates Gena. "My mother put everything on hold in her own life: interests, work, even her health. The kids, husband, and parents came first. Neighbors and friends in need came in next. My mother put herself dead last. I thought that I would never do the same thing, but now I am the glue holding everything together. I became Caretaker Mom, Caretaker Wife, and Caretaker Daughter. Then worked a fifty-hour week. Visits to the gym have disappeared. Most nights, dinner is grabbed on the fly, standing in the kitchen at ten P.M. When I gained forty pounds, I was resentful and angry. I felt completely lost within everyone else's needs."

■ 3. Stress Undereaters

(See Box 3-3 for clinical evaluation.)

There are two subcategories of stress undereating: short-term and lifelong. Anyone, regardless of her usual stress profile, may become a *Stress Undereater* when confronted by severe stress. A lifelong Stress Overeater may experience a tragedy such as the loss of a loved one. In this case the Alarm Hormone is secreted at such high levels that despite a strong genetic and constitutional tendency toward overeating, appetite is suddenly suppressed. This suppression may last for hours, days, weeks, or months. But after some time has passed, a woman will return to her original pattern.

Stress-Resilient women may also experience extreme stress in their lives and may have suppressed eating for a period of time as a result. What is fascinating is that Stress-Resilient women can regroup quickly and without self-destruction, returning to their baseline stress-resilient lifestyle. This is exactly what Non-Stress-resilient women struggle to achieve.

Lifelong Stress Undereaters, on the other hand, tend to see every life event as extreme. For them, the smallest hassle is a crisis of huge proportions. Because of this, their Alarm Hormone remains excessively high all the time. They are always on alert. The light stays on in their head, and they risk serious burnout.

Because the Alarm Hormone is one of the most potent appetite suppressants in the human body, these women live with suppressed appetites and high levels of cortisol. Most lifelong Stress Undereaters are what we refer to as highly restrictive eaters and tend to be obsessively controlling about every morsel they consume.

Typically, anorexics are Stress Undereaters. *Anorexia nervosa* is an eating disorder that reflects a highly overactive stress response. Anorexics have some of the highest levels of Alarm Hormone ever measured in humans. They are rail-thin, with little muscle mass and highly restrictive, often bizarre eating patterns.

As is often the case with anorexics, prolonged elevation of the stress hormones can inhibit the normal functions of the reproductive, immune, and growth systems in the body.

Once a given stressor has been dealt with, Stress Undereaters often indulge in chaotic eating. They roller-coaster between sup-

---

Box 3-3. **Clinical Evaluation: Stress Undereaters**

Alarm Hormone	Very high
Cortisol	High
Eating behavior	Highly restrictive and often erratic; ranges from eating suppression to refeeding after stress
Sleeping pattern	Often agitated sleep; tends to rise early; anxious upon awakening; feels less anxiety as the day progresses
Body composition after forty	Low to average weight, lower than normal muscle mass; minimal meno-pot; high risk for Toxic Weight after the age of forty
Body Mass Index	Low to normal
Physical fitness level	Average to high
Mental and emotional state	Hyperenergetic chronic anxiety, worry, panic; melancholic, or hyper-activated depression; likely to set unrealistic goals; poor regrouper; rigid and highly controlling; tends toward perfectionism
Reward system	Frustrated; unable to achieve sense of pleasure and reward from anything

---

pressed eating and rapid refeeding, and they are always worried about the next stressor. On the surface, Stress Undereaters try to exhibit calm. But inside, they are bathed in high levels of the stress hormone. They feel agitated, anxious, worried, and in need of control. And as a consequence, despite having average weights, Stress Undereaters are at high risk for Toxic Weight accumulation.

Many Stress Undereaters are chronic exercisers. They have discovered that one of the few things that calms them down and relieves anxiety is exercise, usually a vigorous aerobic workout such as running or biking.

Moderate to vigorous exercise results in the secretion of beta-endorphin as well as adrenaline. Beta-endorphin and other proteins are members of the opioid family of human biochemicals, which have a calming and natural anesthetic effect on the body. They are secreted in larger quantities during vigorous activity, and they directly inhibit the stress response, causing a decrease in the Alarm Hormone as well as cortisol. Many people attribute the "runner's high" to this brain chemical. Stress Undereaters are usually acutely aware of its presence during exercise, so much so that they can actually become addicted to the sensation. A Stress Undereater who cannot exercise may experience depression.

Because Stress Undereaters live with constantly elevated levels of cortisol and Alarm Hormone, they become almost numb to their

Case Study—Deborah, Age Forty-two

"As a political fund-raiser, I have a demanding job," says Deborah. "I also have a husband and two sons. My children play every sport imaginable, and we are often all going in six different directions, to soccer, ice hockey, baseball—and of course someone needs to drive them. One morning I had to be at work for an important presentation. My housekeeper didn't show up. It was a disaster. My husband offered to take the kids to school while I went to work and we would talk later in the day. I felt agitated and tense in the car. By the time I got to work, I was shaking and perspiring. I felt so jittery. I couldn't even walk. I thought I was having a heart attack. My partner said, 'Go home and eat something.' In the car on the way home, I thought I would die. I kept pulling over to take more breaths.

"I went to the doctor, and they thought I had a brain tumor. Then another doctor told me I had a panic attack. I knew I was stressed to the max. I was really living on the edge. I'm a runner and tried to do at least twelve miles a week. I'm also a repressive eater. I can go all day long without eating anything and then have a few pretzels for dinner. I wasn't sleeping that well. My husband kept saying 'It's your eating.' He's been saying it for years."

own reward system. They develop a tolerance to experiencing plea-sure or happiness. It then takes higher and higher levels of stimula-tion to experience the reward. That means they require more vigorous levels of exercise to feel the endorphins kick in. Like heroin addicts, they become tolerant of the natural drug's effects and require more and novel ways of achieving the sense of reward. The Stress Undereater's prolonged overstimulation of the reward system even-tually leads to frustration and heightened anxiety as satisfaction is never quite reached.

But because Stress Undereaters have a poor and restricted dietary intake, their constant overexercising compromises their muscle mass as well as their bone mass. Their BMIs are low to average. Poor diet and high levels of cortisol leave them with subnormal strength as well as brittle bones.

By now you should be convinced that stress is an integral and es-sential part of everyday living. Both genetics as well as environment play crucial roles in defining the unique ways in which we respond to everyday stress. I always start my patients on their journey by saying:

> Genetics may load the gun,
> but environment pulls the trigger.

Stress Overeaters as well as Undereaters need to be aware of their tendencies toward self-destructive eating and learn to work with their innate strengths to stop the Toxic Stress and shed their over-forty Toxic Weight. Regardless of your history, realize that you can learn to become more Stress-Resilient.

Now that you are aware of just how your body works under stress, I will show you how to cope better and live well with a healthy attitude and stress-neutralizing eating and physical activity.

Part II
The Three Templates

- **Template One: Stress-Resilient Regrouping**
- **Template Two: Stress-Resilient Nutrition**
- **Template Three: Stress-Resilient Physical Activity**

LIFE STRESS

STRESS—RESILIENT

STRESS—NONRESILIENT

Controlled Stress Response

Uncontrolled Stress Response

NONTOXIC STRESS

TOXIC STRESS

Controlled Eating

Uncontrolled Eating

Nontoxic Weight

Toxic Weight

Fit Mind and Body

Unfit Mind and Body

LIFELONG REGROUPING

Template One
Stress-Resilient
Regrouping

4 Learning the Fine Art of Regrouping

■ The *R* Word

Getting fit and healthy after forty is not a destination. It's a journey filled with trials that test our abilities to live healthfully. Both turbulent and joyous, it's one my women patients have come to embrace through the art of regrouping. And when we shared our thoughts about weight gain and stress, one thing had become abundantly clear to all of them. Eating a brownie would never cure their stress. It would never, as Deb said, "get me where I wanted to go."

■ Plan A and Plan B: How to Be Flexible When Life Doesn't Go According to Plan

■ Stress, Eating, and Relapse: The 72-Hour Recovery Plan

■ The Importance of Self-Care and Balanced Caregiving

But how could Deb and Marcia, Barb and Karen get back on track if they ran into problems coping with issues in their lives and ended up stress eating? I gathered some of my patients together in a group to share their thoughts about this.

"What helps me," offered Deb, "is knowing I have a day or two or three to recover. To not give up or see this as a failure or to completely throw in the towel and say all those negative things that I used to say."

"What *do* you say?" I asked.

"I say it's time to regroup."

The assembled women nodded and laughed. "The *R* word."

Barb chimed in. "It's honoring my feelings and forgiving myself. Saying, 'Yeah, you fell down. You didn't have a good meal or you weren't perfect. It's okay.'"

"I know I'm going to be out of my routine when I travel," said another woman. "But I know that as soon as I return home, I can get back into my routine."

There was a brief silence. Was it really that simple? I wanted them to be honest.

Karen sighed. "Hearing about regrouping is different than the act of regrouping," she said. "I've always had a hard time getting back to my routine if it's interrupted. My mind comes unleashed because I give self-discipline a holiday as well."

I then asked the women to share the reasons they fall off track.

"Life. Work issues. Anything can throw me off course. Sometimes the goal becomes fuzzy. We spend a lot of time saying 'I'm frustrated. I'm sad. I'm fat.' But we don't spend enough time saying 'I'm going to be fit.'"

"There are people who get in the way of your goal. They do not support you, or they sabotage you, or their needs get in your way."

"External factors to which I'm vulnerable and my thought process in not focusing on my goal are the two culprits. They've driven me off course several times and it has taken me months to learn what regrouping means. Sometimes I'm strong in the face of an external factor and I'm okay. But when the two of them meet, I'm in trouble."

"Getting on the scale can ruin a perfectly good day."

How do you begin the journey? It all starts from the neck up. The truth is that a healthy body starts with a healthy mind. Forget the old diet mentality "If only my body were perfect, all my problems would be solved." It's not about squeezing into a size 6 or trying to lose 20 pounds before your daughter's wedding. It's about how you negotiate the maze of everyday challenges. It's about embracing the uncertainty of life and enjoying each new adventure. It's about bending, not breaking. I call this the art of regrouping.

The proof that your mind has a powerful influence over your

body is found in science. At a 1999 meeting of the American Psychological Association, Dr. Barbara Anderson presented results from a continuing study of women with stage 2 and 3 (out of 4) breast cancer who are participants in the Stress and Immunity Breast Cancer Project at Ohio State University. Her groundbreaking study showed that women with breast cancer who were treated with chemotherapy and also received training in relaxation, stress reduction, coping, and social support strategies demonstrated significantly lower levels of cortisol up to eight months after treatment than the group of women who received chemotherapy alone.

The women who received stress-reduction training were also able to tolerate higher levels of chemotherapy. Moreover, these women were shown to have higher levels of an antitumor antibody months later, indicating a healthy immune response to the breast cancer.

"We're finding that stress and distress can be significantly reduced in breast cancer patients," Anderson noted at the conference, "and that these effects are linked to lowering of stress hormones, a stronger immune response, and a better quality of life."

Learning to control your stress hormones will reduce your tendency toward self-destruction and ultimately save your life. This means doing the best you can, working through the day's hassles without mindless eating—standing in a trance in front of the refrigerator, ready to stuff all the problems down with food. Calories are not the cure.

Barbara, a vivacious fifty-five-year-old government policy maker and lifelong Stress Overeater, told me about a revelation that was particularly helpful on her journey toward Stress Resilience. It revolved around her son's wedding. Despite months of planning, things were not perfect. The wedding planner had not followed through and, in fact, had embezzled the monies, resulting in a criminal arrest. The hotel decided to renovate at the last minute. Walls were down everywhere and the pool was a pile of rubble and not a sight for sore partygoing eyes. For the first time in her life, Barbara did not run for the comfort of her refrigerator to numb the pain of these events. She just shook her head, laughed, and said, "What are you going to do?" The wedding went off fine, and everyone had a great time. Barbara negotiated the stresses by *regrouping*.

■ The Plan A Way

The Chinese word for "crisis" is comprised of two symbols, one on top of the other. The first symbol means "danger" and the second "opportunity." In the context of stress and regrouping, the difficulty is the new stress and the "opportunity" is to formulate and follow a contingency plan to resolve the stress.

As His Holiness the Dalai Lama noted in the preface of his book *Ethics for the New Millennium,* "Having lost my country at the age of sixteen and become a refugee at twenty-four, I have faced a great many difficulties during the course of my life. . . . Nonetheless, in terms of my own peace of mind and physical health, I can claim to have coped reasonably well. As a result, I have been able to meet adversity with all my resources—mental, physical and spiritual. . . . Had I been overwhelmed with anxiety and despaired, my health would have been harmed."

The Dalai Lama acknowledges that chronic stress would actually have physical consequences. His extraordinary coping skills sprang from an ability to draw upon inner strength. In essence, his life is a journey of continuing to refine his Stress Resilience.

The art of regrouping is a powerful tool that allows you to capitalize on opportunities that appear in the midst of crisis and to continue a healthy eating and exercise program by offering alternatives to the "ideal" days in your life, which is what I refer to as Plan A. One of my patients compared regrouping to her contingency planning for Y2K. "A lot of what we're doing applies to life skills," she told me one day. "If you can get into this mode of planning for different situations, there's a Plan B and even a Plan C. Have them ready to go into play."

Your contingency plan is Plan B, to be put into effect when everything seems to go wrong. When your best intentions for healthy eating and exercise are thwarted by events outside your control. You need to understand something: you haven't failed. You've just been thrown a curveball. Regrouping is the tool that lets you make a transition between the more controlled routines and rituals in your life and the daily or life-altering stresses that challenge your ability to maintain these regimens. Regrouping permits you to keep your stress hormones at healthy levels, and when those are in check, so is your eating.

Forty-five-year-old Ginnie walked into my office one day and sat down wearily. "I want to be the poster child for the sandwich generation." Over the past six weeks, her mother had been diagnosed with Alzheimer's disease and placed in a hospital, causing her sister to go into a deep depression; her ten-year-old daughter had been diagnosed with attention deficit disorder; and her husband had tripped over the dog, fracturing three ribs, which required her to take him to doctors and care for him at home.

The classic response to such trials for a Stress Overeater like Ginnie is, of course, to eat her way through them. But Ginnie didn't gain a pound.

"I'm getting used to the fact that this is life," she confessed. "And the solutions to any of these problems are not found in my kitchen cabinets." Ginnie is learning how to adapt to the stresses that a rich and complex life presents. That is why I believe that:

Health = Successful Adaptation

There is a movement within tai chi that is referred to as "embracing the tiger." To perform this correctly, you extend your arms out to each side and, slowly, as though gathering all that is around you, bring your hands together, joining them at your abdomen or center of the body. You have embraced your tiger, or all that is life. Then as you integrate the tiger into your being, you push your arms forward, away from your body, bringing them out to the extended position again, a gesture of acceptance toward the inevitability of life's pains and joys. The tiger is a wonderful metaphor for life since it represents all that is powerful, colorful, playful, dangerous, unpredictable, and joyous. And to cope with this tiger, you need a definite plan.

Driving to another state to hospitalize her mother interfered with Ginnie's typical routine. These basic routines include activities—exercise, proper eating, adequate sleep, and moments of meditation—essential to keeping every woman healthy. Under this plan, the stresses of life are manageable.

Plan A = Your Basic Self-Care Done in Your Unique Living
Environment While Stress Is Under Control

Ginnie learned to adapt to her new stresses by developing a Plan B. If she couldn't hop on her home treadmill to walk in the morning, she put on her sneakers and walked around the hospital grounds. While it also would have been easy to resort to chaotic eating (late nights at the hospital, hours in the car), she managed to stay on track.

Plan B = Your Basic Self-Care Done Under Stress

Plan B is a holding pattern, a time when Stress Overeaters as well as Undereaters can learn to "tread weight."

It is realistic to expect that you may not make major strides in removing weight during Plan B. Instead, your objective is to maintain your present body composition while negotiating stress. That's treading weight. It's important to realize that one of the greatest accomplishments in your self-care journey is not to drop weight but to show that you can tenaciously hold on to what you have accomplished under stress. Then you can continue to progress once you have regrouped and returned to your Plan A routine (see Figure 4-1).

Think of how you can apply this to your stress profile. For instance, Stress Undereaters tend to be rigid. They freeze at the first hint of change and cling to Plan A. Undereaters need to practice mental flexibility. This will help reduce their tendency to skip meals and skimp on eating. Stress Undereaters need to tread weight as well, not dangerously drop weight.

When Ginnie proudly announced "My greatest accomplishment is not gaining any weight over a horrendous six weeks," she had learned how to tread weight.

Daily stress can be annoying but livable (you get the flu and stay in bed for a few days). Or the stress can be life changing (death of a loved one), requiring you to reorganize your life and develop a new Plan A.

When she returned home, Ginnie wanted to get back to her old routine as soon as she could. But her daughter's diagnosis was serious and it meant real changes to the family rhythm. Daily tutoring sessions and weekly teacher meetings interfered with Ginnie's usual times for exercise and meal preparation. She was forced to create a new Plan A that would include these adjustments. While it was stressful to help her daughter deal with her learning disability, Ginnie told me she was able to cope as best she could. Her only other option was the "old way," to abandon her self-care entirely, as so many women do.

Try not to cling to your typical Plan A when the need for a con-

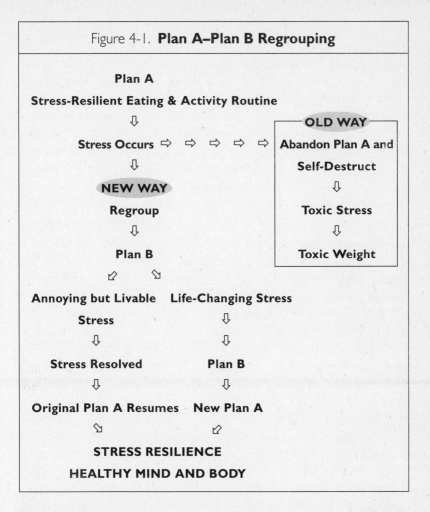

Figure 4-1. **Plan A–Plan B Regrouping**

Plan A

Stress-Resilient Eating & Activity Routine

⇩

Stress Occurs ⇨ ⇨ ⇨ ⇨ ⇨ | **OLD WAY**

| **Abandon Plan A and**

⇩ | **Self-Destruct**

NEW WAY | ⇩

Regroup | **Toxic Stress**

⇩ | ⇩

Plan B | **Toxic Weight**

↙ ↘

Annoying but Livable   Life-Changing Stress

Stress ⇩

⇩ ⇩

Stress Resolved   Plan B

⇩ ⇩

Original Plan A Resumes · New Plan A

↘ ↗

STRESS RESILIENCE

HEALTHY MIND AND BODY

tingency plan becomes obvious. It's perfectly normal to feel intimidated and a little unbalanced by change. Humans are creatures of habit. But there are times in life that simply demand adjustment, and when that happens I want you to understand that everything doesn't have to fall apart.

It's ironic that the old catchword for menopause was "the change." As a woman over the age of forty, embrace this need for change and reevaluate your lifestyle habits. Your reproductive system, body composition, moods, skin, hair, libido—everything is in transition. Everything is changing as you prepare for the next forty years of life.

This is a golden opportunity to create new roles for ourselves, to make our lives richer and more fulfilling. As mind-body specialist Joan Borysenko noted in her book *A Woman's Book of Life,* "Each period of life transition has its own gifts. By her early forties, a woman is poised at the brink of a second puberty, another time of physical metamorphosis critical to her development as a woman."

Women who are not afraid of this second puberty make a relatively smooth transition, emotionally and physically. But all women can be taught the art of regrouping. In fact, most women are masters at regrouping for others. When your child, spouse, parent, boss, or friend needs help with stress in their lives, I guarantee you rise to the occasion. As women, we take pride in rescuing others. But if we try to rescue ourselves, we are left with feelings of guilt and selfishness. *Self* is a four-letter word to so many women. Burdened by attending to the needs of family and work obligations, my patients often say, "I'll get back to eating right when this stress is all over." I gently tell them that it's possible to regroup under these complex responsibilities and become more flexible and resilient and to learn to balance their needs with those of everyone else.

Becoming Stress-Resilient is a process of letting go. Imagine stress as waves in an ocean. As each new wave approaches, instead of standing rigid, trying to withstand the impact, picture yourself lying on your back and floating above the crest of the wave. Try to optimize every challenging situation, thinking, "How can I make this work for me?"

At first, you may not be able to recognize an opportunity. Lance Armstrong, the winner of the 1999 Tour de France, was recovering from surgery and chemotherapy for testicular cancer when he realized he was not going to be able to train in the traditional way for the hill climbs in the Alps. He had lost so much muscle that there was no time to build it up for the race and have the power for hill training. So he and his coach created and designed a special training regimen, or a Plan B, to circumvent this problem. In the end, that training method was to be his signature trademark and proved to be a better way to train for hills than his previous routine. From crisis to glory through Stress Resilience.

Armstrong's story is so inspirational because it provides us with an example of how to negotiate even the most extreme obstacles in our lives to accomplish our goals. I often recite this quote from Henry Ford when I am teaching my patients about successfully adapting to life's stresses, regardless of how impossible the feat may seem: "Obstacles are those frightful things you see when you take your eyes off your goal." Creating your Plan As and Bs throughout life helps to keep that focus crystal clear and transforms obstacles into manageable stresses.

To help you learn to develop Stress Resilience I have written the Stress Resilience blueprint, which will show you how to adapt when stress occurs in your life. You'll always have two choices: to act Stress-Resilient or to self-destruct. You might—like many of my patients—have to work harder than the next person to achieve resilience because of your unique and innate stress hormone levels, but you can do it.

One of the first exercises I give my patients is to examine what happens when a life stress interferes with normal exercise and eating routine (for example, being delayed at work, can't get to the gym, can't eat at the regular time). I ask each patient to keep a journal, logging what her patterns of behavior are when faced with life stresses. These journals are a gold mine of information as patterns of self-destruction become clear. Most important, women learn to identify and stay alert to the *triggers* of their self-destruction. These triggers can be difficult to pinpoint at first.

"I find my goals are deflected by the incident causing stress," said Barb. "I'm trying to overcome really piddling things. I'm trying to learn how to become a master of the situation instead of a victim."

"I still tend to make my schedule around everyone else's, particularly my daughter's," said Jennifer. "I have weeks where I don't care for myself. But that's what I know they are: weeks, not months, not years."

■ Stress, Eating, and Relapse

Over the years, I've had unique experiences helping women learn to manage life's stresses without self-destruction. One woman in particular comes to mind. Whenever she had difficulty dealing with life and ate food inappropriately as a result, she would come to me, ashamed. "Can I still see you? You haven't given up on me, have you? Please, give me another chance!" I was stunned since it would never occur to

Figure 4-2. **Stress Resilience Blueprint for a Healthy Lifestyle**

Stress Undereater	**Stress Resilient**	**Stress Overeater**
Goal: reduce Toxic Weight by calming anxiety	Goal: maintain Stress Resilience	Goal: reduce Toxic Weight by increasing energy/activation
⇩	⇩	⇩
Plan A	Plan A	Plan A
⇩	⇩	⇩
Healthy lifestyle	Healthy lifestyle	Healthy lifestyle
⇩	⇩	⇩
Coping by calming; healthy lifestyle	Coping by balance; healthy lifestyle	Coping by activation; healthy lifestyle
⇩	⇩	⇩
STRESS!	STRESS!	STRESS!

Stress Undereater:

Self-destruct: stop eating ⇩⇧ ⇩⇧ → Anxiety: AH/C high

Go to Plan B: practice resilience through calming ⇩ → AH/C NI

Toxic Weight → REGROUP ⇩ Practice calm AH/C NI

chronic	short-term
⇩	⇩
integrated	resolved

REGROUP ⇩ Original Plan A or Modified Plan A ⇩ Healthy lifestyle ⇩ Continue to practice coping with stress through calming ⇩ Ready for life stresses

Stress Resilient:

Go to Plan B: practice resilience through balance ⇩ AH/C NI ⇩ REGROUP ⇩ Practice resilience AH/C NI

chronic	short-term
⇩	⇩
integrated	resolved

REGROUP ⇩ Original Plan A or Modified Plan A ⇩ Healthy lifestyle ⇩ Continue to practice Stress Resilience ⇩ Ready for life stresses

Stress Overeater:

Self-destruct: stress eat ⇩⇧ ⇩⇧ → Depression: AH/C low

Go to Plan B: practice resilience through activation ⇩ → AH/C NI

Toxic Weight → REGROUP ⇩ Practice activation AH/C NI

chronic	short-term
⇩	⇩
integrated	resolved

REGROUP ⇩ Original Plan A or Modified Plan A ⇩ Healthy lifestyle ⇩ Continue to practice coping with stress through activation ⇩ Ready for life stresses

AH = Alarm Hormone   **C = Cortisol**   **NI = Normal**

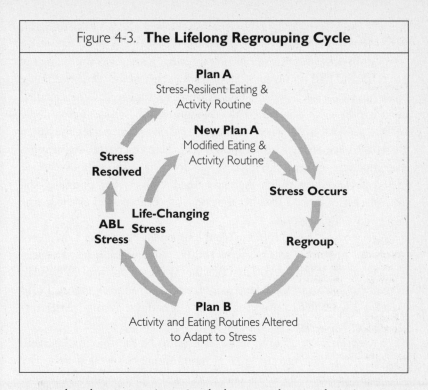

Figure 4-3. **The Lifelong Regrouping Cycle**

Plan A
Stress-Resilient Eating &
Activity Routine

New Plan A
Modified Eating &
Activity Routine

Stress Occurs

Stress Resolved

Regroup

ABL Stress

Life-Changing Stress

Plan B
Activity and Eating Routines Altered
to Adapt to Stress

me to abandon my patient simply because she was learning to regroup and manage stress better.

But I realized that after years of painful dieting experiences, she was convinced she was a failure, not worthy of love. I teach my patients there really is no such thing as failure and that life is a constant state of regrouping requiring patience and perseverance. A perfect example of this is my patient Karen.

A lifelong Stress Overeater, she was 85 pounds overweight when her husband left her for another woman. The extreme trauma caused her Alarm Hormone to skyrocket, resulting in her temporary transformation to a Stress Undereater. With no appetite, she lost 50 pounds in six months. "I couldn't eat. I couldn't swallow. It was devastating." Once the dust had settled, she reverted to her tendency to stress overeat and gained more than 70 pounds. At five feet, three inches, she weighed 212 pounds. Socially, she had withdrawn from everyone in her life, using her weight as an excuse not to go to parties or functions or to the beach in summer. She was also a borderline diabetic, had developed osteoarthritis, which made walking difficult, and suffered from high blood pressure.

Within three months of our first meeting, Karen was following my program and had removed 35 pounds of excess of fat while becoming more physically fit. Then she mysteriously disappeared. When I called her to follow up, she noted overwhelming job stress and said she "would get back to me when it lightened up." Six months later, she called my office back to make an appointment. Her voice sounded frantic. "I completely let go," she said. "I just don't have the willpower."

I asked her how much she had gained. "Thirty-five pounds," she said anxiously. Then I told her that this is to be expected as she learns to navigate life's stresses.

Karen came in and told me what happened. "I had been on a very successful nutrition and exercise routine and walking nearly every day as you recommended. Then one day while on vacation, I decided to participate in the food feasts my friends were indulging in. I told myself I'd get back to my program in a few days. Wrong! After trying to regroup, whatever that meant, I had lost my focus."

A veteran dieter, Karen said, "It used to be that having 'arrived' meant I no longer had to work at maintaining the weight loss. The moment I reached my goal," she said, "I stopped counting calories. Each time I lost weight, the pounds always came back. It was jolting to realize that the process of weight control is lifelong."

For Karen, regrouping required several steps.

- **Acknowledging when she is overeating without being harsh on herself**
- **Deciding to change**
- **Planning what to do instead of overeating (usually getting back to her proven program) and doing what she planned without negotiating or berating herself**
- **Incorporating the experience of a relapse as a positive, no matter what, and determining what the experience has taught her**
- **Accepting that this will come up again and remembering what she learned the last go-around**

The daughter of a controlling man who was obese and died prematurely of heart failure, Karen says at the age of forty-six her time of eating irresponsibly has ended. "Losing weight used to be about my looks. Being fat was ugly. It wasn't until I reached my midforties that losing weight was about my health. The risks are not worth the momentary pleasure of sinfully rich food. But sometimes I feel that I could be tempted again. Will I totally lose control and, if so, will I be able to get back on track?"

That's where regrouping comes in. Losing control does not have to lead to abandoning her goal, as Karen did with her friends on vacation. "This time around, I eat at restaurants and don't shy away from once in a while treats. These things had been forbidden on diets. Instead, I'll try to load up on healthier foods. Rather than eating an entire dessert, I'll split one or take small tastes. I have learned the art of tasting and savoring instead of gulping and overconsuming. By giving myself permission to taste, I don't feel deprived and thus I curb a potential binge."

Once Karen learned the art of regrouping, she had a chance to break the weight gain/loss cycle. She has continued to lose steadily in the last six months, walks seven days a week, and works out with a personal trainer. Physically fit, mentally more Stress-Resilient, and 66 pounds lighter, Karen has humbly recognized that each day of her life is another opportunity to continue to practice and refine her regrouping to maintain what she has achieved. And no, she has not been perfect.

"But I finally did learn the meaning of 'regrouping,'" she said. "Even if it's been a week and I've messed up, it's positively okay. I'm much stronger now. I learned that there is a process in this."

The process that Karen refers to is a basic strategy I teach my patients to help them get back on their Plan A. I call it "Regrouping after Relapse: The 72-Hour Plan." I have learned that once you have lost the momentum of a regular Plan A routine, it is not easy to recapture it, whether you are a lifelong Stress Overeater or an Olympian. Regrouping after having been self-destructive is a painful process. That pain is part of life, since life involves an endless series of regroupings. Say to yourself, "Okay, things got out of control. Now I've got to get back to it."

I have found that if you give yourself three days of "self-destruction withdrawal," you can usually regain that momentum and continue the journey. Why three days? You need time to relearn Plan A, practice it, and let it begin to mentally solidify. You literally need to turn off the negative, self-critical thoughts and get active, jumping into your healthy routine again and seeing the whole process as a natural part of anyone's life.

Of course, you will not have completely regrouped within three days. You are simply putting the brakes on a train that is racing out of control. Once it has stopped, you can proceed with your journey. One of my Stress Overeaters has always referred to food as her heroin, an anesthetic that gave her the only pleasure and comfort in her life. In her self-destructive mode, her momentum was to continually abuse food. As she began the 72-hour regrouping plan, she would refer to each day as "heroin withdrawal day number one, two or three." Eventually, she had counted through thirty before she realized she had successfully withdrawn from her self-destruction and was living her healthy Plan A. She now seeks reward from a rich and fulfilling life, not from food.

So be prepared to revisit the 72-hour regrouping plan as you learn to deal with life stresses. As you become better at this, you will be less afraid of relapses and more adept at getting back to Stress Resilience.

■ Regrouping After Relapse: The 72-Hour Plan

Day #1 Plan your day carefully, arming yourself with the foods and meal planning you need as well as your physical activity. Try to keep this a low-stress day since you are fragile and vulnerable as you emerge from the relapse. It is key *not* to indulge in any type of self-defeating inner dialogues. Just keep your dance card full and stay busy. Stay strong and walk away from opportunities to overeat. Turn your motivation for change into a mantra, a chant to yourself as you face tough temptations to revert to self-destruction. Say it quietly or shout it at the top of your lungs. You need to be reawakened to a self-loving reality. Let any feelings of pain or discomfort pass through you. Don't run from them. See them as a normal and integral part of regrouping. Plan on going to bed early that evening to decrease the likelihood of staying up late and running into problems with late-night eating.

Day #2 Repeat everything you did on day one. You should feel a bit of relief knowing that you made it through one day without significant self-destructive behavior. Again, plan and be prepared. Watch the inner dialogue and fill it with self-affirmations, "You go, girl!" or "You can do it!" instead of self-criticism and condemnation. Keep busy. Reward yourself with a long, hot bath, and try to get to bed early.

Day #3 By now you have two days under your belt. Feelings of accomplishment are beginning to supplant self-hate and condemnation. You are beginning to realize that you will be regrouping countless times in your life and that veering off your self-care is just one opportunity to practice the art of regrouping. You are still vulnerable, so you must try to repeat day two's routine again. But remember to include a special reward for yourself at day's end to recognize your efforts.

> Throughout the three days, try to stay as focused and as flexible as possible. Visualize yourself as a great tennis player ready to sprint for the next ball. You never know just where that ball is coming from, but you're prepared now.

You will revisit this 72-hour regrouping plan countless times during your life. The key is to learn from your past experience. The past, after all, is really good for one thing: learning—good, bad, or otherwise. Whatever the experience, benefit from it.

■ Time to Regroup

Regrouping involves becoming mindful, and that takes a concentrated effort. "I can avoid the pain of my stress by having to go fix something," said my forty-seven-year-old patient Katy. "Cook something. Buy something. Hide from something."

In my experience, women are masters of denying and avoiding their own needs in deference to others. Women have a tendency to jam their calendars with commitments and activities as a form of escape and never put themselves on their own "to do" lists.

Take kids to school
Go to dry cleaners
Lunch with so-and-so
Attend teacher conference
Go to grocery store
Volunteer at church
Help parents with the lawn

Making time for self means working through the feelings of self-ishness and realizing that you deserve joy just as much as the people you continue to serve and please. This is not an easy mental transition. It's downright painful.

Women are often terrorized by the emotional pain that accompanies regrouping. Stephan Rechtschaffen, M.D., founder of the Omega Institute for Holistic Studies, notes in his book *Timeshifting*, "Painful feelings are difficult to face, and we'd rather not feel them if at all possible. So we get busy. We speed up. We substitute action for contemplation. We turn on the television, prepare a meal, do the chores and the Internet, work out, think about anything rather than allow ourselves to be with the feeling we're trying to avoid."

A key to success is respecting the time it takes to plan for your self-care.

After I had appeared as a guest on Oprah Winfrey's show in 1996, she asked me afterward how I define success in weight loss and maintenance. I said that I define it the same way I define success in anything in life—with the four-letter word *time*.

Time is the acid test of your ability to continually regroup, maintain your roles as a mom, daughter, wife, sister, co-worker, friend, community member while staying healthy. Each year the four seasons of your life present you with opportunities to regroup as life throws you one curveball after another. It's a test of how well you can take care of yourself despite these challenges.

A friend of mine proudly announced to me that she had lost 30 pounds in two months by nearly starving herself. "Look at me! I'm a size eight! I was so successful! What do you think?"

"Call me in a year," I replied, "and let me know how you are." Her extreme diet eventually backfired, and she yo-yoed with weight for months. One year later she was 45 pounds heavier, and still gaining.

Time. The ultimate test. And the ultimate luxury. Most women fail in weight-loss programs because they don't give themselves enough time. What they do is give everyone else time.

I will never forget the morning another one of my patients, a lovely, highly accomplished fifty-year-old woman, sat in front of me and showed me her 8" x 11" AT-A-GLANCE calendar. It was literally black with writing, and every line was filled with to dos that involved everyone but her. Doctor appointments for the kids, taking the dog to the vet, meeting her husband for his business party, taking mom shopping, visiting a friend in the hospital. There was literally no room to write in any personal activity for herself. She looked up at me and pleaded, "How am I going to lose all of this weight when I can't even locate myself on my daily schedule?" I sat with her as we went through every day of her week, and she was amazed at how freely she gave away hours she could have spent on her journey to getting fit.

Until a woman learns to treat herself as she does others, she will never be successful in achieving the body and mind that she desires.

Time is a rare and precious commodity for the modern woman. It always involves trade-offs. "Don't make me choose between going to the gym or attending Johnny's thirty-first soccer game of the season." The decision is so difficult, women just slip back into denying their own needs.

At 270 pounds and five feet, nine inches, forty-five-year-old Rebecca laughed when I told her she would have to take time to take care of herself. She exclaimed, "But I do! I call it my 'protein ritual': hair, nails, and teeth." Rebecca was a Stress Overeater most of her life, and her dissociation of mind and body allowed her to live each day without despairing over her own self-neglect. The walls of carefully constructed false realities came crashing down when her doctor shocked her with a new diagnosis of high blood pressure. Taking time to care for herself was no longer about issues of guilt and self-ishness. It was about saving her life.

Ask a woman friend what she'd most like to have more of in her day and she'll say time.

You know the scenario. You're at work and you've just gotten a phone call from your eight-year-old's schoolteacher. Kathryn's got a fever and sore throat. You shift into high gear, making arrangements at work to continue your project in the morning while cramming some papers into your briefcase to review when you can; calling the doctor's office for an emergency appointment; racing out the door; weaving through traffic to pick up your sick child; getting to the doctor; picking up the prescription at the pharmacy; putting Kathryn to bed; and starting dinner. After dinner, you review a few work papers in bed, catch five minutes of the news, and collapse.

Well done, you say. Women are impressive in their ability to regroup and rescue others from the jaws of stress. They repeatedly show the world they can respond with positive force and focus, and regroup in a flash when a life event occurs. We are often given applause when we come through for someone else, especially those close to us. Sometimes, however, we can feel that our efforts go unnoticed or are taken for granted. We are caregivers. It's our nature to give and to keep giving. As women, we frequently give without limits or boundaries. Our standard response for any request for help is yes, without considering our own needs. We worry endlessly about the welfare of others and rarely spend that kind of time or effort on ourselves. That's why I call women *eternal caregivers*. We need to rescue ourselves—from Toxic Stress and the Toxic Weight that will shorten our lives unless we take the time for self-care.

Women often report to me that they begin a new routine of healthy lifestyle habits, happy and fulfilled. Then some life event occurs. It's rarely life threatening. The husband doesn't get a promotion and becomes withdrawn and depressed. The in-law falls and breaks a hip and needs weeks of convalescence. The son begins to drive and gets in a fender-bender. She immediately puts her self-care on hold. Nine times out of ten, the result is weight gain.

One of my patients, Leslie, a successful fifty-year-old journalist with two children in their twenties, once frantically cried out, "I can't get on a treadmill for forty-five minutes! What if someone needed me? What if the phone rang? What if . . ." I was offered a laundry list of at least a dozen "what if" scenarios. I told her that the mathematical probability of a life-threatening phone call coming through while she was on her treadmill at 6 A.M. was low enough that I thought she could proceed without worry. Even if a life-threatening problem did occur, she could respond in plenty of time. Cautiously trusting me, she tenuously began her activity routine in the morning. It took her three months to prove that the earth didn't shake because she took a walk. Five years later, she aggressively defends her alone time, sometimes her day's only time of quiet solace.

Women over forty need all the solace they can get. Perimenopause is in full swing. Your moods are becoming more unpredictable, you may become depressed, your monthly periods are in flux, your memory is shot, you sweat when you sleep, your appetite is off the wall, the fat is increasing, and your waist is expanding. According to Philip Gold, M.D., Chief of the NIH's Clinical Neuroendocrine Branch, "It appears that women are born with stress response systems that are exquisitely sensitive, to enhance their ability to caregive throughout life. But it's a double-edged sword. It also makes a woman more vulnerable to erratic mood swings and this is especially relevant during the perimenopause." The perimenopause, then, is an awakening for so many women. It's a wake-up call that taking time to care for oneself is no longer an option to be dropped. It's a nonnegotiable and integral fact of her life.

Loretta LaRoche, a nationally recognized authority on healing and humor, once noted, "So many women behave like they are the Mothers of Perpetual Responsibility! There's always something you need to be doing for someone. It never ends until you have convinced yourself you deserve to live well, too!"

Caregiving for others while caring for yourself is balanced caregiving: loving, nurturing, and caring for yourself as you do for others. Ginnie learned to do this while caring for her hospitalized mother. She still got that destressing walk in. She still sought out healthy food while she waited in the hospital. Ginnie also learned the importance of balanced caregiving when she enlisted her brother to help with their mother's care. "It's the first time I've let go and let other people take on a crisis. He's doing a good job. And I'm proud of him. If you're dealing with people who need you, you have to be fully charged. The caregiving has to start with me. And the only way to do that is to take time for yourself." It is possible to care for yourself and love and nurture others and is vital in reducing your Toxic Stress and extending your life.

It's no coincidence that women over forty who have managed serious medical problems of a spouse or ailing parents tend to gain weight. There are many overweight and obese widows in my practice, women who have set aside their self-care for years while coping with a sick husband. One in particular, a former athlete and now a fifty-year-old widow, came to see me to find out how to get back into shape. She had given up all but the most perfunctory self-care routines to handle her late husband's prostate cancer. Over three years, she had gained more than 50 pounds. She was newly diabetic and suffered from high blood pressure. She did not know how to regroup. She had no contingency plan, a Plan B. Regrouping also means abandoning perfectionism.

I can't count how many women like Karen have arrived at my office, plopped their bodies down into my Queen Anne chair, and said, "I've been bad. I wasn't perfect." Where did this perfection land mine come from? Did you ever notice when you were growing up that the word "perfect" seemed to be one of the most tormenting controllers of our lives?

I want you to sit perfectly still.
That's perfect!
Oh, look! You're a perfect size 8!
She's so graceful, like a perfect ballerina!
She got perfect scores on her test!
She was always the perfect daughter.
What a perfect mom!
She has a perfect baby!
Your makeup's perfect!
This is the perfect dinner party!
She's such a perfectionist about her house!
She's got a perfect little waist!

Let's see what *Webster's Dictionary* has to say about all of this! "Perfect" comes in three flavors:

perfect (adjective):	"lacking nothing essential to the whole: complete"
perfect (noun):	"flawless, excellent and delightful in all respects"
perfect (verb):	"to bring to completion"

Then there's:

perfectly (adverb):	"in a perfect or complete way"

And, finally, the queen herself:

perfectionism (noun):   "a predilection for setting extremely high
standards and being displeased with
anything less"

Women picked up the message that deviating from some fictitious
standard of excellence constituted failure. This is yet another message that gets in the way of shedding your over-forty weight and finally achieving a healthier mind and body.

Women who are *perfectionists,* I have observed, also take life personally. Too personally. One of my patients, Deb, once told me her
code of ethics for years was "It's all my fault, all the time."

In the end, perfectionism leads to Toxic Stress. The perfectionist
is constantly tormented by the fact that she will never be good (thin,
rich, nice, nurturing, etc.) enough. She doesn't take care of herself because it cannot be done perfectly. She procrastinates because she
fears never being able to live up to her own impossible standards of
excellence.

Dr. Herbert Benson, director of the Harvard Mind/Body Institute, noted in his book *Timeless Healing,* "We harangue ourselves for
not being perfect, for not living life with the panache portrayed in
magazines or on TV. We adulate the firm bodies, we exercise like
zealots or wallow in guilt if we don't, choosing diet shakes over moderation. . . . We aspire to parent perfectly, to juggle flawlessly the demands of work and home, and to have marriages and relationships of
unwavering passion." Benson is telling us that by constantly pursu-
ing unreal goals, we condemn ourselves to a life of frustration, anxiety, and depression. By striving to achieve a mythical perfection, we
are denying our own unique, fallible humanity.

*It is my firm belief that the greatest amount of Toxic Stress comes
from unmet expectations about life.* Messages from society and the
media set women up for unrealistic goals.

- **"If I starve myself today, I expect to lose two pounds by
tomorrow."**
- **"If I skip lunch, I expect to eat lots for dinner without
gaining weight."**

> ■ "If I lose twenty-five pounds, I expect to find a lover/hus-
> band/new job." /

Perfectionists are paralyzed by unmet expectations. Stress-
Resilient women who know how to regroup have realistic goals.

> ■ "If I get more physically active, drop some excess fat, and
> get fitter, I hope to meet some interesting people on the
> hike this summer."

Use the word "expect" for things you have the greatest control
over—those involving yourself. Use "hope" for things over which
you have little or no control, which is everything and everyone else.

> ■ "If I am thirsty, I expect to drink water."
> ■ "If I have Toxic Weight, I expect to change my lifestyle."
> ■ "If I have Toxic Stress in my life, I expect to cope better."
> ■ "If I get off track, I expect to be able to regroup."
> ■ "I hope it's nice weather tomorrow."

Again, the way out is through regrouping.

The antidote to perfectionism is learning to live in the gray zone.
It's letting go of rigidity and replacing it with flexibility by abandoning extremes and learning how to compromise.

The Gray Zone		
White	**Gray**	**Black**
Failure		*Perfection*
Extreme	**Real Life**	**Extreme**
Unhealthy	**Healthy**	**Unhealthy**

There was a wonderful ad that depicted a man with the globe on
his back. It read, "The Earth weighs 30 trillion tons. Isn't it about time
you let it go?" Living in the gray zone allows you to achieve Stress Resilience, to relieve you of the burden of carrying all that weight.

Substitute the perfectionist diet speak of old with your own
speak. We'll call it woman speak. Give it your name! Deb speak!

Try it out using the familiar and demoralizing language of diets:

Toxic Stress	Realistic Adaptation to Life
Diet Speak	*Woman Speak*
I wasn't perfect.	I did the best I could under the circumstances. I will strive to do better tomorrow.
I want to be a perfect size.	I want to achieve the best fitness I can.
I'll be perfect tomorrow.	I did my best today, and I will try to do better tomorrow.
I cheated and wasn't perfect.	I deviated somewhat from my normal routine. I made adjustments and I'm okay now.
I didn't eat perfectly.	I didn't eat appropriately, but I will make adjustments and eat better next time.

Finally, women are the most avid readers and students of health and wellness books, newsletters, and magazines. Most women know the basic essentials to achieve their health goals. However, I have noticed that many women read and think about health but frequently don't act on it. These women are thinkers. *Ponderers.* Frankly, we, as women, like to ponder, to go over details, to wonder. As I mentioned in Chapter Two, women's brain circuitry is unique in that, in comparison to men's, it tends to contemplate and analyze the whys and wherefores of situations in our lives. On the one hand, all this thinking is wonderful, as we work out the details of our lives: children's educational directions and mapping out how to care for our loved ones. But, like caregiving, thinking needs to be done with balance. The balance is generated by action. Thinking about taking a walk doesn't make you fitter but actually taking the walk does.

Forty-nine-year-old Cathy was a classic example of a pondering, perfectionist eternal caregiver. At five feet, five inches and 200 pounds, she was at high risk for diabetes and heart disease, both of which ran in her family. She had plenty of Toxic Weight on board and was feeling less and less energetic every day. As part of her program, I told her to start taking forty-five-minute walks, either using her treadmill or outdoors in her neighborhood. Then I watched as she struggled through the process.

She pondered: When to walk? If I walk in the morning, I have to get up earlier and go to bed earlier. Can I do that? What about my favorite show at night? Can I give it up? I'm not really a morning person. Can I change? What if I get up in the morning and I feel too tired to walk? If I walk at night my husband will feel abandoned if I'm not there to care for him. I get home from work right before dinner, so how do I wedge it in anyway? Can I get to work earlier, use my time better to leave earlier? But then my fellow office workers might think I'm slacking off since I usually stay with everyone until 6:30 P.M. every night and they might not like me as much. I ache every time I walk. My knees hurt. I should only walk outdoors when the weather is perfectly cool, not hot or cold. On and on it went.

She came back a week later never having walked. It was a beautiful spring day and she was wearing casual clothes and comfortable shoes. I asked her whether or not she had thought about going out and enjoying the weather and the gorgeous blossoms. "I thought about it," she replied, "but by the time I wanted to do it, there was no time."

I asked her when was the last time she had taken a walk by herself, just to enjoy getting out. She couldn't remember. Knowing that she lived nearby, I said, "Why don't I show you some wonderful walking paths while we talk about your self-care issues?" She stood up and said, "Let's do it." I let her lead the way. Halfway through the walk, Cathy's face was flush with pink and a radiant smile had replaced her frowning and stiff upper lip. "Wow! I had forgotten how good this feels. I feel like I could conquer the world!" she said. She liked it so much that, of her own accord, she made plans to walk the next day. From thought to action. And the payoff was a vibrant sense of wellness!

I have observed that women get hung up in an endless mental struggle with past and future obsessing. Their inner dialogues often begin with "If only I had" or "What if." Rummaging around the past and worrying about the future occupy valuable time that should be spent productively doing self-care in the present.

■ Regrouping for Life

Over the years, I have watched many women become more Stress Resilient. These women have noted that the same resilience that helps them stay fit and healthy has also made it possible to cope with stresses. They have learned to practice lifelong regrouping to stay healthy (see Figure 4-3). Stress-Resilient patients have shared with me some of the most important tools and techniques that helped them continue to succeed. Consider these useful options while refining your personal Plans A and B.

- **Create a support system. One patient's greatest support system is her dog. (Yes, she jogs with him.) Another's is women in her book club. Support systems are nonjudgmental. People who support your efforts must be there for you as you regroup time and again.**
- **Tap into your spirituality. At the Harvard Mind/Body Institute, Dr. Herbert Benson has demonstrated that people with the strongest belief systems had greater rates of survival and optimal healing from surgery than those with no belief system.**
- **Joy and laughter reduce stress hormones. Dr. William Fry, a Stanford University psychiatrist, noted that children laugh more than four hundred times per day. This decreases to fewer than a dozen times daily for adults.**

Scientists have been studying the effect of humor on the body for years. By learning to find humor in life you can actually

- **Get a great workout—laughing for at least ten minutes is equivalent to rowing for 100 strokes**
- **Reduce stress hormones**
- **Increase beta-endorphins, which relax you as well as help contain the stress response**
- **Boost your immune system by activating the production of key white cells**

Developing a realistic wit and humor, then, is one of the most valuable tools to keep you on track as you begin your journey.

It's always helpful to have an itinerary for any journey. Something I have convinced my patients to do is keep a private journal. I ask them to write down when they feel stressed and to make an immediate association between eating and the event as it occurred during the day. In the journal, many women see for the first time the triggers of Toxic Stress, which maintains a lock on their excess body weight. It is important to make associations between what and when you feel stimulated to eat as you attempt to cope with daily stresses. The journal is your physical and emotional log book, and it is a critical part of your journey and a wonderful help in learning to regroup.

Here are a few helpful hints to begin your journal:

- **Buy a special journal that is as unique as you are. I personally recommend *A Woman's Book of Changes: A Guided Journal* by Tools with Heart.**
- **Find a private space to relax in as you record your thoughts.**
- **Do not censor yourself. Learn to write freely, expressing your emotions as you see fit.**
- **Write in the journal every day, even if it's a single word only. By doing this, you create a ritual that you'll honor.**
- **At the end of every week, look back at what you have written and ask yourself, "What have I learned?"**

When I recently saw Johari she told me, "The more I use my journal, the more I like it. It's a useful tool, and I can take it with me. It has space for three main meals as well as snacks. I record the time, the amount, and what I am feeling. The major thing for me is knowing what I'm eating. There are days I think, 'I really don't want to write this down.' And you write it down saying, 'I know what I did.' Pizza. Carrot cake. Chocolate candy. I know it's a setback, but it's not going to kill me."

I asked her to define regrouping as it pertained to her journey. "I think regrouping depends on your personality and whether you really have the exercise and eating discipline ingrained. After years of free-falling," she told me, "it takes a while before this takes hold."

"Sometimes I'll be writing it down, and I'll say 'Four really not great days in a row,'" said a patient one day. "I can't figure it out right away, but it helps keep me focused. If I didn't have a journal, I'd be thinking, 'It's only been two days I haven't done well.' Writing it down is logging it in on paper. You can't lie to yourself."

"Getting off track is breaking a promise to yourself," one of my patients told me. "And that's the worst kind of promise to break."

So now you've been introduced to the First Template: The Fine Art of Regrouping. Next you will learn how to apply the principles of regrouping as well as the science of stress eating to your daily, over-forty nutrition and physical activity.

As you begin your journey, let Naomi's voice comfort you as you regroup and learn to inhabit your own life.

> *Today I give birth*
> *to the woman in me*
> *who has waited so long*
> *to be acknowledged.*
> *I welcome myself to the world*
> *and I will not forget again*
> *that service to self is a worthy task.*

> —From "Entitled" by Naomi

Template Two
Stress-Resilient
Nutrition

5 Navigating the CortiZone

Body image: nothing can boost a woman's confidence or send her self-esteem plummeting like stepping on a scale or glancing into a mirror. Concern about body image is probably the number one anxiety among women.

Trying to achieve an unreasonable weight is the most frustrating exercise for women. And the Toxic Stress of years of dieting has left them on a perpetual roller coaster of self-love and self-hate. Closets become metaphors for how well a woman is coping with her life. By the age of forty, most women's closets resemble department store retail racks, with clothes which range in size from "thin" to "fat." And as a woman progresses through the perimenopause, elastic waistbands replace belts as Toxic Weight replaces her premenopausal waist.

- The CortiZone: The Danger Time for Stress Eating

- High-Quality/Low-Stress Eating

- When to Eat: Barbara's Story and the Daily Food Pyramids

One of my patients walked into my office after having lost her first 10 pounds and was celebrating by wearing a new outfit. Without realizing what she said, she asked me, "Does this stress make me look fat?" Stunned, I realized she wasn't aware of what she had just said. I thought to myself, "Even dressing has become associated with Toxic Stress!"

Even after achieving higher levels of fitness and shedding excess fat weight, many women cannot believe their own reflections. Fat heads linger in fit bodies. Many women who set physical perfection as a goal are convinced that a certain body type will bring them happiness. *"If only I were thinner . . . taller . . . smaller . . . had a waist . . ."* In the perimenopause, the new player is the Toxic Weight of the ever-expanding waistline.

■ The Toxic Stress of Dieting

If you were born between 1944 and 1959, you belong to a generation of women who came of age along with the diet industry. As children, we were told to clean our plates and be mindful of the starving children in Third World countries. Later, we were presented with the ideal figure of womanhood: a 90-pound, wide-eyed British waif whose very name, "Twiggy," foreshadowed a wave of crash diets and slimming products. The rounded curves of the fifties woman were supplanted by thin limbs and bony chests, and self-esteem was calculated by scale weight.

When did all this start? Originally, eating was tied to a healthy lifestyle. The Greek word *diaita* was first used to describe one's manner of living. The English translation came to mean not only the manner in which we eat but what we usually consume. The modern connotation suggests that our daily fare should be subject to limitation. And now the word is generally used to describe a selection of food geared specifically to "losing weight." The French call it *la régime,* meaning a strict regimen adhered to for a short period of time to get quick results.

Today, it appears we've come full circle as we struggle to return to healthy lifestyles. As veterans of the diet wars, women are beginning to change their perspective and view "diet" and "thin" as four-letter words. *Fit* is in. Becoming mentally and physically healthy is the new goal.

To achieve this healthier lifestyle, women over forty have to put into perspective years of messages from the diet industry that have tried to convince them that there was something wrong with their appearance and seduce them with quick and easy solutions.

In the early 1930s, a doctor in Chicago began promoting "Dr. Stoll's Diet-Aid, the Natural Reducing Food" in beauty parlors. Women were told to stir one teaspoon of his miracle elixir (milk chocolate, starch, whole wheat, and bran) into one cup of water (11 calories total) and drink it for breakfast and lunch.

That same decade, the "Grapefruit Diet"—also known as the Hollywood Diet—was introduced. It included a few vegetables, tiny amounts of protein, and lots and lots of grapefruit, which was said to contain a special "fat-burning" enzyme. Nonsense. I could put you on the "Hydrangea Diet" (same foods, replace the grapefruit with the plant) and you would lose weight because of the limited amount of calories. Trust me. There is no fruit that burns fat, least of all grapefruit. Grapefruit juice is a diuretic. You'll lose water weight, not real weight.

Many of my patients have also tried the "Cabbage Soup" diet. Cabbage is a vegetable. It has no miracle weight-reducing properties. You *will* lose weight if you eat nothing but vegetables. All you are doing is cutting calories with your favorite substance *du jour,* whether it's cabbage, celery, or yucca.

But women bought these "miracle" diets because there was no other real information coming from the medical community. While scientists were studying nutritional issues, who was going to fill in the information gap? The grapefruit people. The chewy chocolate reducing people. (Remember Ayds?) Retailers, diet gurus, and entrepreneurs looking for a quick buck. In the 1960s and 1970s, "diet doctors" were medical practitioners who worked from a repertoire of therapies that included diet pills. In 1970, 8 percent of all prescriptions in this country were written for amphetamines, 2 billion (including refills) of them specifically prescribed for weight loss.

Little good medical information came out of this new "diet industry," only hype and false hope—and continuing dieting stress.

The Tab years. Fresca. Sego. Metracal. We lived on instant "slenderizing" drinks and frozen grapes, starch blockers, lobster for breakfast or nothing but fresh fruit before noon. I once came across something called the "Twenty-first Century Diet," which consisted of goose and quail eggs for breakfast and three green peppers for dinner. There are so many extreme diets which found popularity that it's hard to list them all: Bananas and Skim Milk Diet, No-Sugar Diet, Rice Diet, Potato Diet; all dairy, no dairy, all carbohydrates, no carbohydrates. And let's not forget the Popcorn Diet!

Clearly, most everyone would love to be thinner and they are willing to pay for it. By 1999, the sales of commercial diet programs, foods, books, appetite suppressants, hospital weight-loss programs, health clubs, surgery, and spas had reached more than $30 billion a year. According to recent findings, on any given day, at least 20 percent of the population in America is dieting to lose weight.

What has been the result of this national investment in seeking slimness? Americans have steadily become fatter and more unfit than any time in history.

In 1997, the Centers for Disease Control and Prevention (CDC) announced that, for the first time in history, there were more overweight and obese adults than average-sized adults in America. Sadly, one in four children is now overweight or obese as well. At the same time, physical fitness levels have plummeted. Currently, more than 30 percent of adult American women are obese (defined as being 20 percent or more above ideal body weight) and 25 percent of men are obese. And the results of a 1999 study by the American Cancer Society of one million men and women showed an unquestionable association between a BMI over 26 and disease and death.

The CDC findings also noted that the most unfit and overweight segment of the population was the baby boomers. Women currently in their forties and fifties represent a significant majority of this population. And the old standby diets are failing them.

Diets fail because no one can live on them for long. Dieting is one of the most psychologically and physiologically stressful things a woman can do to herself. Dieting leads to Toxic Stress.

How? Psychologically, dieting distracts women's search for self-esteem away from their personal and professional achievements and focuses it on their physical appearance. Dieting fosters a dissociation between mind and body. The very act of getting onto a scale is a case of attention being diverted away from the body and onto a piece of metal with numbers. A dieting woman is caught up in following strict rules or food plans that don't feel good but that she tolerates for the short term. Her mood and her world revolve around the success of The Diet.

Dieters become obsessed with their weight and appearance (often to the exclusion of other interests in their lives) and this may trigger feelings of isolation and depression. Poor self-image and self-esteem follow dieting failures. On the flip side, a successful diet may act as a "high" for a dieter and keep her locked into a pattern of further weight loss to capture the same attention for her achievements. With no energy for anything or anyone else and their attention devoted to food and eating, they are literally *"prisoners of weight"* (POW). They live in fear of the next meal, the next holiday family gathering, the next office party. They avoid certain foods, skip meals, try every new diet that comes along. POWs are lifelong dieters.

Statistics have shown that a small number of people manage to lose 10 to 15 percent of their weight and keep it off. The constant lose-gain cycle eventually leads to a constant sense of self-hate, frustration, desperation, and failure.

These feelings are carried throughout each day. They become the heavy mental burden of chronic, relentless anxiety, and sadness. They become Toxic Stress. When Toxic Stress is ever-present, the stress hormones are constantly elevated. As we have seen, chronic exposure of body organs and tissues to high levels of stress hormones leads to

- **Abnormal cravings and eating behaviors**
- **Impairment of the body's immune, reproductive, and growth systems**
- **Mood disturbances, such as irritability, anger, and depression**
- **Poor memory and concentration**
- **Profound lack of energy**
- **Serious medical conditions, including heart disease and diabetes**
- **Weakened muscles and bones**
- **Decreased metabolism**
- **Poor sleep**

But Toxic Stress isn't the only reason dieters can't lose weight. Chronic dieting actually makes you fatter and less able to remove excess fat weight. How? Let's look at how this evolves over time.

A twenty-year-old, five-foot, five-inch woman gains 60 pounds through overeating and lack of exercise. Once 140 pounds, she now weighs 200 pounds. She has never dieted before. She panics and starts a starvation diet of no more than 1,000 calories per day. She does not exercise. Her initial body composition assessment is as follows:

Starting Body Composition
Body fat: 38%, or 76 pounds
Muscle mass*: 55%, or 110 pounds
Body weight: 200 pounds

(*Gross approximation of muscle mass, excluding the weight of bone, water, and hair.)

She sheds 50 pounds rapidly over three months but cannot tolerate the starvation any longer. She starts to overeat again and gains back to her original scale weight of 200 pounds. (In reality, most dieters gain back more than they lose, but for the sake of argument, let's assume she went back to her beginning weight before dieting.) Her body composition is now

Body Composition After Diet 1
Body fat: 42%, or 84 pounds
Muscle mass*: 51%, or 102 pounds
Body weight: 200 pounds

(*Gross approximation of muscle mass, excluding the weight of bone, water, and hair.)

Fed up with her weight, she repeats the diet cycle again, starving and losing 50 pounds and gaining back to 200 pounds. But she notes that it is harder to shed the weight the second time. Her body composition is now:

Body Composition After Diet 2
Body fat: 46%, or 92 pounds
Muscle mass*: 47%, or 94 pounds
Body weight: 200 pounds

(*Gross approximation of muscle mass, excluding the weight of bone, water, and hair.)

Do you notice a pattern? With each dieting episode, she strips precious muscle mass from her body and replaces it with more fat weight. *For every pound of muscle mass lost* (8 pounds after the first diet and a total of 16 pounds after the second), *she has decreased her metabolic rate by 35 to 50 calories.* Let's see how this adds up:

After Diet 1:	8 lbs x 35 = 280 calories per day
	8 lbs x 50 = 400 calories per day
After Diet 2:	16 lbs x 35 = 560 calories per day
	16 lbs x 50 = 800 calories per day

She is losing the power to remove her excess fat. Her muscles, which are her "generator," are dwindling and cannot burn as many calories. Now, if she doesn't consume 560 to 800 fewer calories per day, she'll gain weight. That's a lot of calories, essentially the equivalent of one meal! If she once consumed 2,000 calories to maintain a weight of 200 pounds, she now has to cut her consumption to 1,200 to 1,500 calories just to remain at 200 pounds and not gain any more weight! If after the second diet she goes back to consuming 2,000 calories a day, she will gain weight.

1 pound fat = 3,500 calories

If she consumes an extra 560 calories per day, she will gain 1 pound of fat every six days; consuming 800 calories, she will gain 1 pound of fat every four days. In other words, dieting is a slippery slope: the more restrictive you are, the harder it becomes to lose weight.

The bottom line is that the years of chronic dieting gone through by the majority of women over forty have left them metabolically cooler, burning calories much less efficiently, gaining weight with ease, and desperately struggling to remove the pounds of excess body fat. This causes tremendous chronic mental anguish, Toxic Stress, as women watch their weights soar and their bodies deteriorate, along with the energy needed to live a rich and full life. Physically, after forty, not only does the weight continue to pile on from incessant dieting, but it now accumulates inside their abdomens. *The dedicated dieters of the 1960s are now the perimenopausal women of the 1990s,* who are carrying the accumulated stress of years of dieting and tortured body image around their waist as Toxic Weight, which threatens much more than their self-esteem: it encourages disease and early death.

■ Going Against the Grain

Every year, nutritional scientists make discoveries that can help us eat in a healthier way. For instance, one important discovery was the association between the daily consumption of the micronutrient selenium and a decrease in the risk for colon cancer. It has also been found to be important for women over forty to consume B vitamins and folate to decrease the risk of heart disease.

At the same time, consumers are being exposed to new thinking about how to eat. For instance, the past ten years have witnessed the emergence of diets that manipulate specific nutrients. For example, heavy emphasis has been placed on the reduction of carbohydrate intake in deference to fat and protein intake. This is actually an old concept, which I believe was reborn as a consequence of an epidemic of carbohydrate overconsumption, especially refined, processed sugars. I believe that the main problem stemmed from the advent of the "fat-free" revolution of the 1970s and 1980s, when a greater awareness of fat's role in heart disease and obesity fostered a sense of fat phobia. Americans did indeed ingest fewer fat calories, but replaced them with uncontrolled portions of carbohydrate calories, resulting in greater total caloric intake and a worsening obesity epidemic in America. Also, carbohydrates are unique in that they are easy to access, a real "grab and go" food in a world of fast-paced anxiety about time. Most snack items are chock-full of low-quality carbohydrates.

But let's not throw the baby out with the bath water. Everyone can agree that Americans need to minimize or avoid the consumption of refined, processed sugars. Many people refer to these as the "bad" carbohydrates. These include foods that contain sucrose, or table sugar. Candy, cookies, and dessert items come to mind. But these "bad" carbs also include the white, refined starches as well—breads, rice, and pasta foods, which have been processed and have lost their healthy fiber and nutrients, and have literally been stripped of their color, from the natural browns of the whole wheats to white. This processing removes valuable vitamins and minerals and leaves you with a foodstuff that acts just like a lump of sugar or a candy. That is, these refined sugars raise your insulin levels so high that you end up with a voracious appetite, making overeating and bingeing a common occurrence.

The bath water, therefore, is the refined, processed sugar. The baby, however, includes fruits, vegetables, and the healthy, unprocessed starches. These high-quality carbohydrates provide essential, immune-boosting nutrients for you. These are what so many people refer to as the "good" carbohydrates.

Fruits and vegetables contain valuable plant chemicals called phytochemicals, which include nutrients, vitamins, and antioxidants. Some diet books recommend the elimination of many fruits and vegetables simply because they may raise the blood sugar level to varying degrees. But scientists have found that many phytochemicals are powerful agents that help prevent as well as treat many medical conditions, including heart disease and cancer. Great caution should therefore be exercised before eliminating any of this nourishment.

The same goes for the dark, unprocessed starches. White, processed starches have been depleted of their valuable fiber and healthy nutrients. That fiber is essential to maintain the integrity of the intestine's lining and provide rapid transit of bowel contents. Societies that have the highest ingestion of fiber and grain also have the lowest incidence of colon cancer.

Some of you may already be panicking. You may be afraid of the starches in general because you notice that some of even the high-quality unrefined starches may induce a big appetite. That's normal and you just need to work with foods that don't induce the tendency to overeat.

Foods affect people differently. One person may have a candy and walk away untroubled by appetite. Another may eat that same candy and be left with a terrible appetite for more, and then overeat. This occurs with any food. One of my patients found that the healthy, whole wheat pastas always caused an uncontrollable appetite, even when eaten in appropriate portions. She has lived well for the past two years with no pasta in her life. Instead, she has replaced that starch with healthy portions of brown rice, which she has never had problems with. Fruits can also be troublesome. Grapes are loaded with natural, simple sugar that can cause heightened appetite problems in some people.

A few words to the wise about how to approach this whole carbohydrate issue. First, just because a particular fruit or vegetable is scientifically known to increase your blood sugar somewhat does not mean it will induce an uncontrollable appetite in you specifically. My point is that rather than ban all fruits, vegetables, and whole unprocessed starches, try them out to find out which seem to cause problem appetites and which don't. Once you know which are user friendly, then you can include them in your daily nutritional plan without worry about overconsumption.

In summary, here are some key points to remember when thinking about how to eat carbohydrates for healthy nutrition:

■ **Minimize or avoid foods with processed, refined sugars, which include table sugar, candy, pastries, as well as the processed (white) starches such as pasta, rice, and bread.**

■ **Maximize your exposure to *unprocessed* starches as well as fruits and vegetables. Strive for five (servings of fruits and vegetables every day)!**

■ **Remember that even when you eat healthy foods, too much of a good thing can put the weight on! Later in this template, you will learn about how to choose a woman-sized portion and avoid overeating at meals.**

■ **Use trial and error to find out which foods are *bingeables*. These are foods of which you cannot have just one, and you usually end up eating the whole thing. Avoid these foods as they are nothing but trouble.**

The bottom line is that rather than avoiding all grain and cereals, it is much smarter to include them in appropriate servings and portions (as we shall see in later chapters).

■ The CortiZone

Recall from Chapter 2 that your stress hormones peak early in the morning, at about 6 to 8 A.M. This means that your Alarm Hormone, cortisol, and adrenaline are at their highest levels in your bloodstream. It is during this time that you feel most energetic, attentive, focused, and able to concentrate. By midmorning, your stress hormone levels slowly begin to decline, and by midafternoon you can actually feel the drop in energy and mental concentration. This usually occurs at about three to four o'clock. Biologically, your body is preparing you to rest and, finally, sleep, after a long day of activities. Finally, your stress hormones reach their lowest levels during sleep, allowing you to relax fully. By 2 A.M., your stress hormones are beginning to increase, preparing you to awaken again in the early morning.

This stress hormone biorhythm had a very distinct evolutionary purpose. It was geared to awaken us in the morning and keep us alert, energized, and ready to meet the challenges of the day. It allowed for optimal physical performance, as well as maximal focus and attention for the purpose of survival. It is natural and normal to feel less energy as the day progresses. Consuming the final meal of the day in the early evening and optimally going to sleep by eight or nine o'clock is in sync with the normal biorhythm of stress hormones.

Overeating in the late afternoon and evening is one of the biggest culprits behind stress-induced weight gain in women over forty. I refer to the hours between 3 P.M. and midnight as the "CortiZone," the time when stress hormone levels plummet and mindless, unfocused, stress driven eating dominates, guaranteeing weight gain, especially in women forty and over. It's almost as if your taste buds were linked to your stress hormone biorhythm. During the CortiZone hours any person is at great risk of stress-induced eating. As focus, concentration, and mindfulness decline, fatigue sets in. Instead of recognizing the decline in energy as a natural daily event, most people fight it. Desperately seeking energy, they gulp coffee and eat food high in sugar and other stimulants in the hope of resurrecting their energy.

In today's busy daily life, we no longer live by our natural stress hormone biorhythm. Instead, just at the time of day when we should be allowing ourselves to begin to rest, we start up yet another day's worth of errands, projects, activities, and challenges.

Isn't it interesting that most people don't stress-eat first thing in the morning? That's because, regardless of your stress profile, your stress hormones are at their peak and keep you more alert and focused in the morning. You feel hopeful, ready to face daily challenges. Women get busy writing their "to do" lists and charge ahead with the day's activities.

By midafternoon, a woman in her forties begins a particularly stressful phase of her day. As the CortiZone begins, she often faces carpooling, project deadlines, business travel, rush-hour traffic, attendance at school functions, business dinners, children's homework to help with, and countless domestic errands. All of these require attention, focus, and concentration, just at the time of the day when the stress hormones that control these are declining. Frustrated and anxious, perhaps unconsciously so, women turn to food for activation as well as anesthesia from the pain of having to bear this kind of burden later in the day. By dinnertime, it is no wonder that women ofttimes feel like rewarding themselves for surviving yet another day. Many women tell me that the only time of day they truly have to themselves is late in the evening, after the rest of the family has retired to sleep or engage in other activities. Late-night, after-dinner eating is a common habit of exhausted and overburdened women who are seeking peace and solace and who want to enjoy the momentary pleasure and relief of their favorite anesthetic, food.

Each of the stress-eating profiles deals with the CortiZone differently. As you can see in Figure 5-1, a Stress-Resilient woman follows the natural curve of the cortisol biorhythm, respecting its declining levels as the day progresses and planning around the fatigue and potential for mindless eating later in the day.

The problem begins around 3 to 4 P.M. At that time, the stress

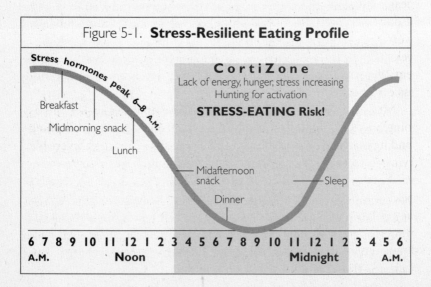

Figure 5-1. **Stress-Resilient Eating Profile**

Stress hormones peak 6–8 A.M.

Breakfast
Midmorning snack
Lunch

CortiZone
Lack of energy, hunger, stress increasing
Hunting for activation
STRESS-EATING Risk!

Midafternoon snack
Dinner
Sleep

6 7 8 9 10 11 12 1 2 3 4 5 6 7 8 9 10 11 12 1 2 3 4 5 6
A.M.   Noon   Midnight   A.M.

hormones are at approximately half their morning level, and most people are beginning to feel tired, as if they are losing their edge. This is the beginning of the CortiZone, when a woman begins to feel very vulnerable to stress eating. The CortiZone extends all the way through midnight. But it is often how a woman handles the beginning of the CortiZone that establishes how she will handle it later.

■ Stress Overeaters and the CortiZone

Stress Overeaters set themselves up for problems later in the day by either eating too lightly at breakfast (a piece of toast or a bagel) or skipping breakfast altogether. Lunch is often either skipped or skimped on; a yogurt, a small container of cottage cheese, or a bowl of soup is the typical lunchtime fare. By the beginning of the CortiZone, most Stress Overeaters are feeling starved.

Stress Overeaters tell me that they are "great" until the mid- to late afternoon, when they seem to lose their "willpower" and blow the day's good intentions with stress eating. What happens? When our cortisol levels plummet, we feel tired and in need of rest. Instead, we're at work or busy with home activities or on the run somewhere, and rest is not an option. Also, it's been at least three hours since a meager lunch, and our hunger is on the rise. Stress is high at this time of day. Work pressures as well as family commitments often create overwhelming anxiety. Desperate to stay alert and active, women seek energy through coffee and food to stave off the hunger. As concentration and focus wane with the declining levels of cortisol, mindless eating takes over.

Marj, a Stress Overeater, refers to these episodes in her life as going into "fog mode" or a trancelike state. She doesn't recall piling vending machine fare into her mouth as she sits at her desk feverishly trying to meet another deadline, and yet eating brings a sense of reward and pleasure. Midafternoon is a time when Stress Overeaters seek food pleasure to help neutralize the mental pain of the stresses they must continue to endure to get through the day. The more Marj perceives the stresses on her as horrific, the more stress eating she indulges in. Stress Overeaters are often found *asleep at the meal*, engaging in mindless stress eating throughout the CortiZone.

Kerry, another Stress Overeater, used to come home in the late afternoon after a long day of working, carpooling, and grocery shopping and find herself standing in front of the refrigerator, door open, just staring into the brightly lit shelves filled with wonderful things. Her husband watched her do this one night and told her that her frozen, glazed look reminded him of a deer caught in headlights. She had no memory of walking in the front door, taking off her coat, and heading for the refrigerator. She was in a stress trance, drained and exhausted and searching for a fix, a reward. She managed to pull herself back to reality when her husband jokingly hung a pair of sunglasses on the refrigerator door. From then on, playing along with the joke, she wore them whenever she opened the refrigerator door. This example is typical of someone who is "asleep at the meal."

Midafternoon is very challenging for a Stress Overeater. Recall that Stress Overeaters have an abnormal stress response, in which there is an imbalance of stress hormones throughout the day, with more cortisol than Alarm Hormone. This leads to a heightened vulnerability to stress-induced appetites when stress seems uncontrollable. "Stewing and chewing" becomes a serious problem during the CortiZone.

Once stress eating has started, it sets up a mind-set of hopelessness and continued eating. When she finally gets home, the Stress Overeater continues to snack or binge through dinner and frequently up to bedtime. As her stress hormones continue to fall further, preparing her for sleep, the Stress Overeater feels unable to muster the energy and concentration to handle the stress. Instead, once again, she uses food to anesthetize herself from the pain of coping with chronic stress. In essence, Stress Overeaters' eating patterns don't seem to follow the food pyramid. Instead, they eat according to the Stress Overeaters' pyramid (see Figure 5-2).

■ Stress Undereaters and the CortiZone

Recall that Stress Undereaters perceive most daily stresses, which could be viewed as ABL stresses, as crises that induce chronic anxiety. Because they awaken with higher-than-normal levels of stress hormones, they often wake up early and feel agitated. Vigorous exercise, such as running, often quells that agitation since beta-endorphins (as

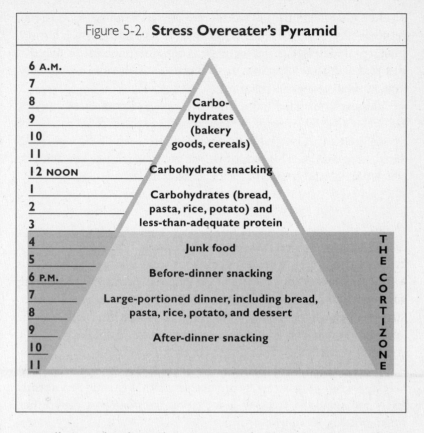

Figure 5-2. **Stress Overeater's Pyramid**

6 A.M.
7
8   Carbo-
9   hydrates
10   (bakery
11   goods, cereals)
12 NOON   Carbohydrate snacking
1   Carbohydrates (bread,
2   pasta, rice, potato) and
3   less-than-adequate protein
4   Junk food
5
6 P.M.   Before-dinner snacking
7   Large-portioned dinner, including bread,
8   pasta, rice, potato, and dessert
9   After-dinner snacking
10
11

THE CORTIZONE

you will see in the Physical Activity Template) are potent neutralizers of the stress response. Without some way to control the early morning anxiety, it is difficult for chronic Stress Undereaters—who are at high risk of Toxic Weight because of chronic stress—to perform their daily functions well.

While not necessarily healthful, morning eating for the Stress Undereater is often controlled and simple, as is the lunchtime meal. Overeating is not a problem, since the Stress Undereater's stress hormone profile shows an imbalance favoring more Alarm Hormone than cortisol, the opposite of the Stress Overeater. The Alarm Hormone is a potent appetite suppressant, and too much of it will lead to reduced appetite and caloric intake.

Absorbed by the day's crises, the Stress Undereater rarely eats in the afternoon and therefore still maintains stress-induced appetite suppression. Interestingly, many Stress Undereaters may actually feel somewhat less agitated as the day progresses, since stress hormone levels are decreasing, reducing the sense of mental frenzy to a more comfortable level. The dinner meal is often minimized or skipped, and thus valuable nutrients are not consumed because of the controlled, restrictive eating pattern.

This overcontrolled and restrictive eating is physiologically as well as psychologically stressful for the Stress Undereater. This pattern of eating often leaves her feeling mentally agitated, physically weak, and unbalanced overall. This unhealthy behavior constitutes Toxic Stress, which will inevitably lead to the deposition of Toxic Weight.

■ Stress Resilience and the CortiZone

Although Stress Overeaters are at greatest risk of weight gain during the CortiZone, each stress profile needs to learn to eat more healthfully throughout the day. Learning how to work with cortisol's natural biorhythm is imperative to achieve good health and avoid Toxic Weight.

The goal is to achieve Stress Resilience by modifying your daily habits to keep your stress hormones as close as possible to normal levels and avoid the Toxic Weight that results when they are left elevated and out of control.

Here are some helpful hints to allow you to successfully navigate the CortiZone:

- **Prepare by planning. Be realistic. If you know that the day is going to be a bear, arm yourself with a daily eating plan, as well as ways to blow off the stress steam throughout. Plan to escape and take a walk whenever you can.**
- **Know what you are going to eat for your midafternoon snack and dinner. Arm yourself with healthy food during the CortiZone (you will learn more about this in the next chapter). Without planning, you leave yourself vulnerable to overeating during the CortiZone.**
- **Stress Overeaters need to keep their eating plan simple and straightforward, avoiding too many options and steering clear of freestyle, "anything goes" patterns of eating.**

■ **Stress Undereaters need to add regularity to their daily routines by eating small meals even when they don't feel like it. It is physiologically stressful for the body to habitually experience severe caloric deprivation followed by erratic feedings.**

■ **Acknowledge the physiologic fact that you will become mentally and physically tired after 3 P.M., and that such a decrease in energy is normal. Try to organize your day so that you have fewer stressful projects and intellectual challenges after 3 P.M. If you have no choice and you have to handle a stressful project in the CortiZone, break it up into miniprojects that can each be seen as doable and less stressful.**

■ **Beware products that promise activation or calming. These "rewards" come at a very high price. Out of desperation, both Stress Overeaters and Stress Undereaters often seek to modulate their stress through caffeine, nicotine, medications (over-the-counter diet pills), alcohol, and food. All of these options can get you into trouble, especially since they are usually consumed to excess.**

■ **The easiest way to both calm and activate yourself is through physical activity. Stress Overeaters and Stress Undereaters will both benefit from doing consistent physical activity. Aside from keeping your body composition optimized by burning excess fat and building muscle, exercise controls your stress hormones as you will see in the Physical Activity Template.**

■ **Learn to regroup after an onslaught of stress by using your head as well as your body. This is where forms of meditation such as the Relaxation Response (see Appendix B for additional mind-body resources, specifically the Harvard Mind/Body Institute) come in handy! Your body can also help rescue you through the activation of beta-endorphins when you get up and move it vigorously (e.g., a brisk walk for 30 to 45 minutes). The endorphins inhibit the stress response and bring the stress hormones back into the healthy range.**

The CortiZone is a fact of every woman's life. Navigating the CortiZone safely and without self-destructive stress eating is the goal. Stopping the stress-fat cycle through well-planned and stress-neutralizing eating is essential to achieving Stress Resilience.

■ High-Quality/Low-Stress Eating

After age forty, your body begins to change. That includes your metabolism, hormones, bone structure, skin, hair, waistline, and even appetite. In fact, many women in their forties tell me they have strange new cravings for sweets and other foods they never wanted a decade ago. What's going on?

Many women who have never given up their childhood eating habits seem genuinely shocked when I tell them that at the age of forty they simply cannot eat the old June Cleaver pot roast and mashed potato supper every night, especially if they're coming home from a board meeting at 10 P.M. with a roaring appetite after a stressful day.

Our appetite is also linked to our culture. Food is a loving, nurturing, pleasurable substance. Just the smell of something warm and familiar can trigger all sorts of pleasant memories. Turkey roasting on Thanksgiving. Hot cinnamon-laced cider on a snowy Christmas day. The smoky haze from the barbecued burgers on the Fourth of July. Hot dogs at the ballpark. Any of these smells, wafting over us, can trigger pleasant associations.

There is no reason a woman cannot enjoy these enriching foods from her childhood. The difference is that after the age of forty, women must understand that *the quantities they eat of most foods must decrease as the quality of eating increases.* This means that instead of gulping and overconsuming, a woman must now learn to *taste and savor.* What does this mean? This means that instead of eating an entire box of fat-free cookies, a woman should savor one or two *real* cookies that she purchased as a special gift or treat for herself. She will feel physically and psychologically more satisfied and fulfilled after the real cookies. There is no deprivation, just appropriate, balanced eating.

Women need to honor their eating patterns and requirements. We are not men, children, infants, teenagers, or aged. Yet we are conditioned to eating portions best suited to others, and more often than not it's Man Food. Even restaurant portions are typically man-sized. Hungry Jack pancakes. "Manwich" sloppy joes. Chunky soup known as The Manhandler. Hungry-Man frozen dinners. Hero sandwiches. Big Macs. Burger Kings. The list goes on. *We need our own Woman Food.*

I don't mean more dieting and deprivation. I mean real food, geared toward a woman's need for protein, carbohydrates, whole grains, fruits, and vegetables—and, yes, the occasional treat.

If you want to shed fat after forty, you must believe that *you are different now that your body now has different needs.* You've done the diets. You've accumulated Toxic Stress. Substituting Woman Food for Stress Food will help you begin the journey toward overcoming these obstacles.

Remember, this book is not about steely willpower or swearing off every treat. The minute you say to yourself "Okay, that's it. No more potato chips for the rest of my life" is the second you begin craving them. Johari realized that it was unrealistic to "pretend that you're not going to eat your favorite food[s] again. If you feel the urge, go with it and get over it." You must begin to learn the art of tasting and savoring. It's knowing how your body works. What your woman's body needs to operate at its highest energy level. You must choose jewels, not junk; quality, not quantity.

As one of my patients says, "Invest in yourself and the food you want."

Your metabolism has undergone its third decrease in three decades, and you do not require the same number of calories as you did in your twenties and thirties. The average forty-year-old man's resting metabolic rate is at least 400 calories higher than yours, which means that if a man requires 2,000 calories a day just to remain at the same weight, you need only 1,600 calories. In addition, your muscle mass is smaller. Muscle decreases in size if it's not used. Over the age of forty, chances are you are no longer playing college sports or carrying babies around the house. And if you don't use it, you lose it.

Which means you can no longer afford to waste one single calorie on large quantities of "cheap" or Low-Quality/High-Stress foods. By these I mean foods high in calories and low in nutrients. This includes all of the fat-free dessert items, which are loaded with refined sugar (sucrose) and contain little nutritive value. These Low-Quality/

High-Stress foods are physiologically stressful since they require your sugar-processing hormone, insulin, to go into overdrive to handle the large excess of sugar. High levels of insulin stimulate a voracious appetite, which may precipitate overeating and bingeing. When insulin exceeds a specific threshold level in your bloodstream, your appetite kicks in and all the willpower in the world won't help you.

For example, if you have the option of eating an apple or a fat-free cookie, which do you choose? If you choose the fat-free cookie, you simply pop it into your mouth, and as the food settles in your stomach, it immediately releases extremely high levels of refined sugar, which shoots into your bloodstream and stimulates a raging appetite. Suddenly, you find yourself craving the entire box of cookies and you are consumed with guilt and anxiety and—after the box is gulped, self-hate and disappointment. The grand result is that you have induced both physiological as well as psychological stress, which, when repeated again and again, becomes Toxic Stress. And, as you know, the accrued Toxic Stress is transformed into excess Toxic Weight around your waistline.

What if you had eaten the apple instead? You would have taken time to chew it and swallow it, unlike simply popping the cookie in your mouth. An apple is easier to taste and savor. Because it has bulk and fiber, it occupies more space in the stomach, expanding the stomach walls, which then transmit a message to the brain that you are becoming full. As the apple is broken down in the stomach, it releases into the bloodstream a natural sugar, fructose, which does not require insulin for metabolism in the same way refined, processed sugars do. Therefore, after eating the apple, insulin levels do not rise significantly and further appetite is not stimulated. Now you know why the last thing you want after eating an apple is another bag of them.

Essentially, a fat-free cookie is a Low-Quality/High-Stress food and the apple is a High-Quality/Low-Stress food. High-Quality/Low-Stress food is Woman Food.

Under stress, we have a tendency to eat Low-Quality/High-Stress foods because they are often easy to access and cheap to buy and require very little preparation. The price you pay for gulping Low-Quality/High-Stress foods is that they can cause your insulin levels, cholesterol levels, and/or blood fats to soar. The guilt and anxiety we may feel when we eat these foods adds psychological stress to the eating process. Many women would tell themselves, "I ate junk . . . I'm a failure." My patients only initially feel this way—not after a couple of months.

To destress the eating process psychologically, it is imperative to keep it simple. I subscribe to the ethic of *Keep It Sublimely Simple* (*KISS*). This means *how* and *when* you eat must not increase your stress. So many of the women I work with have a tormented relationship with food. Most would rather not think about eating at all, succumbing to chaotic, grab-and-go nutrition. By keeping the eating process simple, a woman is less likely to obsess and further her mental stress about eating. Simple, straightforward rules of the road allow her to relax more and concentrate on her life, not torture herself over choices and options. Once you've streamlined your eating plan practicing KISS, you will be less likely to search out Low-Quality/High-Stress foods. Indeed, one of my patients declared that "getting fit took less mental energy than living fat."

A cup of chamomile tea is guaranteed to destress you. So is a serving of fruit or vegetables or whole wheat pretzels. Cereal products with little or no refined sugar are also fabulous High-Quality/Low-Stress foods. They give you the carbohydrate calming effect without the insulin kick that refined sugar can have.

As a rule, any food that doesn't cause your insulin to shoot up rapidly through the appetite threshold is High-Quality/Low-Stress food. But to thrive on High-Quality/Low-Stress foods and to survive the daily challenge of the CortiZone, you must be prepared. You cannot rush home after a busy day and expect to eat well if you haven't prepared.

Vince Lombardi, the winningest football coach in history, once said that the secret of success in winning a game was not predicated upon how much you wanted to win. Instead, the team that usually won was the one that was *willing to do what it takes* to win. Work, not wishing, accomplishes the win. Planning how and what to eat is what it takes to keep the fat off.

Therefore, if you fail to plan, you plan to fail—which is why so many women over forty succumb to inappropriate eating during the CortiZone. According to a 1999 survey by *Food Technology* magazine, when a cross section of men and women was asked at 4 P.M. what they were going to eat for dinner, 60 percent of the respondents had no idea.

It's great to be spontaneous, but, let's face it, most of us tend to overeat at night if we haven't planned. Having the right ingredients on hand, whether at home, in your office, or in your car, is no accident. It's important to shop for yourself, keeping a small stash of healthful treats in your car and stocking your office refrigerator with the right things.

What can you do about it? You must begin to shop with High-Quality/Low-Stress foods in mind. One of my patients actually makes a separate grocery run every week—no kids in tow—to stock up on her own foods. As she goes down the aisles, she chooses what's right for her. Her basket may include tofu, fresh fruits and vegetables, hearty, low-fat canned soups, pita bread, cottage cheese, all-fruit preserves, yogurt, low-fat cheeses, rice cakes, low-fat tortillas, canned tuna, chicken or salmon, high-protein cereal, oatmeal, string cheese, frozen fruit sorbet, reduced-sugar canned fruits, and veggie burgers. This way, even when she can't buy fresh fish or lean meat for dinner, she is always prepared. When hunger strikes, she is well stocked with her own choices and won't be tempted by Low-Quality/High-Stress foods.

If you don't buy it, you can't eat it. That means I also want you to plan tasty treats into your own grocery shopping. There should be a balance of 80 percent High-Quality/Low-Stress foods, with a buffer zone of 20 percent treats. This includes Woman Food portions (one serving) of *real* ice cream or one or two *real* cookies or a shared restaurant dessert as an occasional treat (once or twice per week). By planning your treats, you avoid the old diet deprivation mentality because the new rule is that you can eat most foods if you simply know how and when to do so.

Do you happen to like ice cream? You're not the only one. My advice is to plan to eat it and make it high quality. Plan to have a small scoop of the very best, real ice cream as an occasional treat. Feel the creamy texture on your tongue. Allow yourself to enjoy the moment and you won't find yourself in that stress trance, standing in front of the freezer ready to demolish the whole pint of fat-free junk. My patient Helen's treat of choice is Ben & Jerry's S'mores Low Fat Ice Cream. She refers to it as a "lifesaver" and incorporates it into her eating plan.

However, even the best-prepared woman can be overwhelmed with feelings of hopelessness under extreme stress, especially during the CortiZone. We know that stress increases our intake of snack-type junk foods, particularly at this time. Our intake of meal-type, high-priority foods—fruits, vegetables, meats and fish—declines. Stress challenges our healthy eating.

All women, regardless of their stress-eating profile, selectively increase their consumption of Low-Quality/High-Stress foods when they are anxious. Why is it that *stressed* spelled backward is *desserts*?

- **Low-Quality/High-Stress foods taste good. Remember, sugar and fat are the primary "fight-or-flight" fuels. Under stress, as your cortisol levels rise, you will preferentially select foods high in these nutrients. If you were preparing for an actual *fight* or *flight* in response to stress, you would need a calorie-dense food that would supply energy quickly. But since our stress today is from the neck up, the extra calories are not needed or used and end up being stored as fat. In addition, high sugar and fat combinations such as desserts and candy are usually packed with flavor. There's an instant "hit" to the taste buds. Unfortunately, these foods are also high in calories, which means you get an overdose of calories in a very small amount of food.**

- **Low-Quality/High-Stress foods require little to no preparation. Ordering a pizza and thawing out a cheesecake is simpler than taking the time to make dinner. The classic "drive-buy" foods found in fast-food restaurants also fall into this category. Many women, when fatigued, go into a "stress trance" and mindlessly reach for these foods without thinking.**

- **Low-Quality/High-Stress foods can affect brain chemicals. One example is disordered serotonin metabolism, which has been noted in eating disorders. Serotonin inhibits stress eating by controlling the Alarm Hormone. In the perimenopause, when estrogen declines, so does serotonin, resulting in cravings for foods that increase concentration, mainly carbohydrates.**

- **Low-Quality/High-Stress foods are typically "bingeable" foods that can be eaten in large quantities in a single sitting. These foods, classically, do not come in single-serving packages. Instead, they come in family-sized bags, boxes, or cartons. The bingeables include crackers, chips, cookies, cake, and ice cream. A food is bingeable if you cannot stop eating after one average serving.**

One of my patients came to me one day, distraught. She had a craving for jelly beans every day at 4 P.M. and binged on handfuls of them at that time. One well-meaning co-worker had gone out and surprised her with a three-pound jar of the candy to keep on her desk. A typical Low-Quality/High-Stress food, jelly beans were her "tranquilizers" during the day—except that the insulin jolt made her even hungrier, leaving her more vulnerable to the CortiZone crash. I taught her a neat trick: when I asked her which flavor she liked best, she couldn't tell me. She had always just gulped them all down. Instead, I taught her to taste and savor the flavors she enjoyed the most. She came back the next week and reported that in fact, after experimenting, she really liked only two flavors. She then went to a gourmet shop, purchased only those two flavors, and kept a single serving of these flavors in a plastic bag, which she enjoyed each day at four o'clock. This became her treat, didn't lead to a binge, and allowed her to gain control over her mindless snacking.

■ Barbara's Story

But how can you control what happens under Toxic Stress? Unfortunately, that can be the downfall of even the most intelligent woman. Let me use Barbara as an example to illustrate what women typically do as they enter their forties, not realizing what the stress hormone cortisol is doing to their bodies and why being prepared for the CortiZone every day is so crucial. Her story shows what happens when stress and poor planning collide.

You may remember Barbara from our group discussion. She is the one who identified stress eating as "the itch you can't scratch." Perfectionism is her stress trigger. Recall that when she first came to me, Barbara was thirty-nine and weighed 180 pounds. She is five feet, four inches tall. She grew up the beautiful blond teenager who perceived her weight gain as the ultimate fall from grace.

Barbara's a lobbyist, and although she's not on any medications, she has high cholesterol, borderline hypertension, lack of energy, fatigue, and mild depression. Obesity runs through three generations of Barbara's family. Her maternal grandparents were overweight or obese and have been all their lives. Her mother has always had a weight problem. Her brother is overweight, and her sister Marcia, who was obese, is now a healthy weight.

Barbara is married, but not happily. She has two children, a nine-year-old daughter and a thirteen-year-old son. She does some aerobic activity, including occasional walks for exercise. Barbara had always been pear-shaped, but now she is noting that her waist size is increasing. She feels softer and flabbier all over, especially in her upper body. "What am I doing wrong?" she wondered, exasperated.

When we first met, I asked her to give me a typical daily schedule.

7:00 A.M.: Barbara wakes up and has coffee while she zips through the paper. She showers, tends to the kids, and grabs a bagel and orange juice to eat in the car as she drives to work.

8:00 A.M.–12:30 P.M.: Barbara races from one meeting to another, both inside and outside the office. Sometimes she begins to feel weak. She is very hungry before lunch and says she often feels shaky.

12:30–1:30 P.M.: Barbara takes a client to lunch and tries to watch what she eats, despite her ravenous appetite. Usually she restrains herself and orders only a small salad with chicken because she's on "a diet." Eating light, she says, makes her feel "good," if sometimes deprived. At lunch, she is a determined calorie counter.

3:00–4:00 P.M.: Nonstop meetings and telephone interruptions. Barbara says she often feels sleepy and less energetic after lunch and starts craving something sweet to "pick her up." She tries to refrain from eating at this time.

4:00–5:00 P.M.: Barbara is stressed with work and is seriously hungry. She hits the vending machine for a candy bar. She feels guilty for "cheating" on the diet. This guilt makes her feel hopeless. Then she succumbs to a few cookies in her office. She continues to forage for food, but nothing seems to satisfy her hunger.

5:00–7:00 P.M.: Barbara tries to finish some loose ends in her office before heading home or out to a business dinner.

7:30 P.M.: Barbara takes a few clients to dinner. They order and have a drink and appetizers of crackers and cheese; the entree doesn't arrive until 9:00. She orders exactly what the men do—restaurant-sized portions of steak, potatoes, pasta—as well as a portion of rolls or bread. Occasionally, she will have a glass of wine as well. She often indulges in dessert. Since she had such a light lunch, she doesn't feel guilty eating a "healthy" dinner. (After all, she's always eaten dinner late. And she deserves it after her stressful day!)

She then heads home. On nights when she doesn't eat out, Barbara is an after-dinner snacker, sometimes eating right up until she goes to bed around 11 P.M. Snacking on her favorite "fat-free" cookies is a way to "pick herself up" and allow her to stay up later and get more work done.

Diagnosis: Stress Overeater at risk for Toxic Weight.

Like the majority of Stress Overeaters, Barbara consumed the majority of her food in the CortiZone, during the late afternoon and evening, as shown in Figure 5-3. This is a virtual prescription for

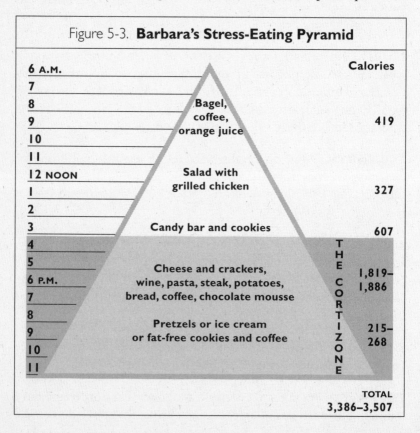

Figure 5-3. **Barbara's Stress-Eating Pyramid**

Time	Food	Calories
6 A.M.		
7		
8	Bagel,	
9	coffee,	419
10	orange juice	
11		
12 NOON	Salad with	
1	grilled chicken	327
2		
3	Candy bar and cookies	607
4		
5	Cheese and crackers,	1,819–
6 P.M.	wine, pasta, steak, potatoes,	1,886
7	bread, coffee, chocolate mousse	
8	Pretzels or ice cream	215–
9	or fat-free cookies and coffee	268
10		
11		

THE CORTIZONE

TOTAL
3,386–3,507

weight gain in women over forty. If you're like Barbara, go to Figure 5-4 and fill in your average daily eating.

During our first sessions, I convinced Barbara that she needed to invert her Stress Overeater's pyramid and prioritize consuming at least 65 percent of her daily calories before 5 P.M. This means that her breakfast, midmorning snack, lunch, and midafternoon snack would now constitute the majority of her caloric intake for the day. Barbara should concentrate on eating more High-Quality/Low-Stress foods in Woman Food portions.

I introduced Barbara to the concept of moving between Plan A, which is her basic daily routine, and Plan B, which constitutes any threat or challenge to Plan A. In essence, Barbara was going to learn how to regroup when her more peaceful and less stressful self-care schedule was under siege from the day's activities. Following are

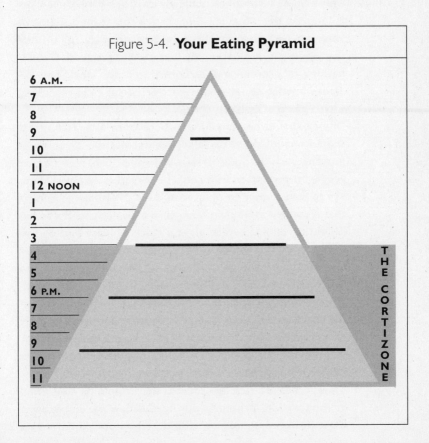

Figure 5-4. **Your Eating Pyramid**

basic principles for her—and every woman—to follow. The details of these will be presented in the following chapters.

✓ Make sure to eat a healthy breakfast no later than 9 A.M. even if it means placing a bowl of oatmeal on your dressing table to eat while you put on your makeup.

✓ Eat a small midmorning snack approximately three hours after your breakfast. This could be a piece of fruit, a small fat-free yogurt, or one or two pieces of low-fat string cheese. The only exception is if three hours after your breakfast is lunchtime.

✓ Try not to eat lunch later than 1:30 P.M. Lunch should include a healthy balance of High-Quality/Low-Stress protein, fat, and carbohydrates (see Chapter 6 for details).

✓ Three hours after lunch is usually the beginning of the CortiZone. At this time, it is imperative to eat food that provides you with High-Quality/Low-Stress energy at a time of day when you are becoming hungry and fatigued. Combinations of protein and carbohydrates are ideal. This includes low-fat or fat-free yogurt or cottage cheese, along with a piece of fruit.

✓ Dinner should be started anywhere from 6 to 7:30 P.M. It should include soup or salad, vegetables, and a source of protein, such as poultry, lean red meat, fish, legumes, or veggie burger. Mixed fruit could be served as a dessert item.

✓ Try to have dinner completed by 8 P.M. My favorite saying is that *if you eat after eight, you gain a lot of weight!* Try to finish eating dinner before eight o'clock at least four to five days per week. If you must eat dinner after eight, eat lighter and eat before you go to dinner—or, the later you eat, the lighter you should eat. For instance, if you had your midafternoon snack at 4 P.M., three hours later, at 7 P.M., repeat the snack so that your 8:30 or 9 P.M. meal consists primarily of vegetables, a small amount of protein, and fruit, if desired.

✓ Women over the age of forty do not require dense complex carbohydrates (pasta, bread, potatoes, or rice) after 5 P.M. These foods are rich fuel sources that should be consumed in moderation, primarily during the day. At dinnertime, these starches should be considered as occasional treats (once or twice a week, in small portions). The goal is to debulk your dinner of the dense calories from complex carbohydrates. These foods, which were once considered a staple, should now be an infrequent dinner treat.

✔ Water should be consumed throughout the day. Often when we think we're hungry, we're actually thirsty. Eight eight-ounce glasses should be drunk during the course of the day.

✔ Plan your treats and remember to slow down, enjoy, taste, and savor your High-Quality/Low-Stress food.

✔ Plan to eat High-Quality/Low-Stress foods during the time of the CortiZone. Mindless eating of Low-Quality/High-Stress foods during the CortiZone occurs when meals are not planned.

✔ Dispose of all fat-free desserts and snack items in your kitchen. They are riddled with Low-Quality/High-Stress re-fined, processed sugars.

✔ Each week, plan to have a treat or two of a Woman Food portion of a dessert or entree item you typically would not consume. Take time to enjoy, taste, and savor these treats.

✔ Be careful of alcohol. It adds 100 calories per glass of wine to your meal. Cocktails have two to three times that amount! Also, after one glass of alcohol, a woman's ability to stick with High-Quality/Low-Stress foods can be impaired. I would rec-ommend alcohol consumption no more than once or twice a week, with one glass of wine at each occasion.

✔ Typical restaurant portions are man-sized. At lunchtime, remember to eat only half of any restaurant portion of starch and try to eliminate it at dinner. At lunch, one piece of bread from the bread basket is appropriate. At dinner, hand the bread basket back to the waiter. Remember: the later you eat complex carbohydrates, the more weight you gain.

✔ Fight for your right to consume High-Quality/Low-Stress food in appropriate woman-sized food portions wherever you may be eating. Be assertive when ordering.

Barbara began to apply the above checklist to her life. Her clients didn't mind eating dinner at an earlier hour; they wanted to get home, too. I formulated for Barbara an exercise prescription, as you will see in the Physical Activity Template. Exercising every day revved up her metabolism, diminished her need to seek activation from food, and gave her more energy. Her 4 P.M. snack prepared her for the CortiZone, and she stopped hitting the vending machine. Eating appropriately during the day actually helped protect her during the CortiZone by leveling off her hormones.

Barbara's "diet" has been replaced with healthy, appropriate eating that she can live with. If she deviates from her plan on occasion, she doesn't see it as the end of the world. She understands that she made a choice when she had a treat and no longer perceives the conscious indulgence as a form of failure or cheating.

Women become stressed about food because they have a deprived mind-set, which made Barbara feel angry at the supreme injustice that others can enjoy foods she can't. Food choices then begin to terrorize. The truth is, we can eat anything we want, as long as we do it appropriately.

Barbara no longer rates her day and eating by the notion that she's "good" if she eats next to nothing. She has snuffed out the deprived mind-set. Most important, food is no longer the anesthesia she uses to dull the pain of life's stresses.

Stress can completely destroy all your planning and commitment when it comes to appropriate eating, especially during the CortiZone. Barbara—a chronic dieter—usually entered that time of day totally unprepared. She did not understand that Toxic Stress during the CortiZone encouraged mindless stress eating.

Basically, we reversed her stress-eating pyramid pattern so that eating in the later part of the day, or the CortiZone, was deprioritized. Barbara's new Plan A (see Figure 5-5) eating routine was now:

6:30 A.M.: After walking on the treadmill for forty-five minutes, Barbara showers, dresses, and sits down to breakfast with her children when she can. She has oatmeal with fresh fruit or cinnamon or cereal with sliced banana, plus orange juice and milk.

10:00–11:00 A.M.: Barbara takes a short break from work sometime during this hour. She sits at her desk and while on the phone or working at the computer eats a container of low-fat yogurt and a few crackers she has brought with her from home. This will tide her over until lunch. She no longer feels shaky before lunch.

12:30 P.M.: Barbara goes out for lunch. She orders salad, a portion of lean meat or fish, and a small serving of complex carbohydrate: pasta, rice, baked potato, or bread. Sometimes she has a serving of fruit as well, along with lots of water.

4:00 P.M.: As Barbara enters the CortiZone, she is no longer ravenous, but she knows that she must eat something to prepare her for what's ahead. She takes a brief break from work and has a cup of cottage cheese and fruit or soup and crackers and more water. She feels satisfied and continues her work. Fatigue is no longer a problem.

7:00 P.M.: Barbara leaves work and goes to dinner with clients. She orders salad, lean meat, and a double order of vegetables. Iced tea has replaced cocktails. Occasionally, she orders fruit for dessert.

Most eating after 8 P.M. has ceased. This is a sacred template she follows.

Figure 5-5. **Barbara's Inverted Pyramid: Plan A**

Time		Calories
6 A.M.		
7	Oatmeal with cinnamon, orange juice, skim milk	270
8		
9	Low-fat yogurt, crackers	321
10		
11		
12 NOON	Salad, grilled chicken breast, brown rice, fresh fruit plate	345
1		
2		
3	Soup, crackers	150
4		
5		
6 P.M.	Salad, lean meat, vegetables, iced tea	240
7		
8		
9		
10		
11		

THE CORTIZONE

TOTAL 1,326

Remember that this is an example of one woman's daily habits. Your needs will be unique. What we have presented are guiding principles. Barbara has found that having lean meat once, perhaps twice per day, rotating with fish as an entree, has left her feeling more satisfied and less apt to binge on sugars and fats. Most women make the mistake of eating too little protein and instead overcarbing with Low-Quality/High-Stress foods. A balance is required.

Barbara has noted interest in experimenting with vegetarianism, which is growing in popularity in the United States. One of the best sources of information to teach you how to get the protein you need without fish and meat is the Vegetarian Resource Group in Baltimore, Maryland. More information is available in the Nutrition Resource List in the appendix. Take a moment and fill in your new Plan A (Figure 5-6).

But what happens when stress hits? Obviously, none of us lives in a permanent bubble of calm and everything going according to schedule. What happens when the baby-sitter doesn't show up, the treadmill is broken, we have to go out of town, or we simply don't have the time or energy to plan and shop for our High-Quality/Low-Stress foods?

We regroup! Our routine under less stress (Plan A) is adapted to the stress (Plan B). I taught Barbara to develop a Plan B for whenever significant stress challenged her regular routine. Rather than doing what most women would do, which is to cling desperately to Plan A and then panic when it doesn't work, adapting to the stress is the answer. Plan B is based upon the principles of Plan A. This means that you will still have breakfast, but it may not be at home, in the comfort of your kitchen.

Barbara began to learn to formulate her Plan B (see Figure 5-7), which might include the following scenario:

7:30 A.M.: Barbara forgot to set the alarm, and the alarm clock doesn't go off. Everybody oversleeps. There is no time for breakfast at home. She grabs a yogurt, an apple, and a cup of coffee and consumes them in the car on the way to work.

10:00 A.M.: Barbara is hungry. But she's in a meeting and can't leave. She reaches into a briefcase, unwraps a small energy bar, and munches on it during the coffee break. The meeting goes on until 11:30. She drinks water with the energy bar and feels fine.

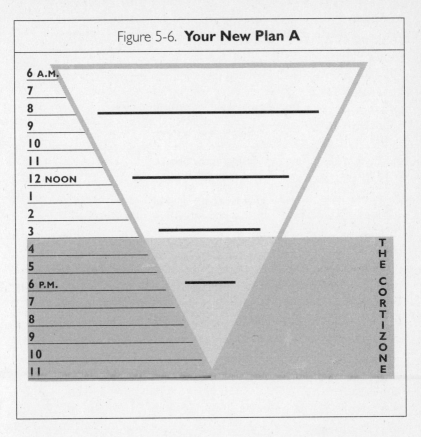

Figure 5-6. **Your New Plan A**

12:00 P.M.: Barbara is under a project deadline and needs to work at her desk. Rather than skip lunch, she orders in a cup of soup, a turkey sandwich, and fruit. She works through lunch and feels better.

3:00 P.M.: She missed walking on the treadmill that morning, so Barbara brought her sneakers to work. She tells her secretary she's "running" an errand and goes out for a brisk thirty-minute walk. Her metabolism goes up, and she feels revived.

4:00 P.M.: Barbara looks in the office kitchen and finds the bag of low-fat string cheese she had brought in for the week. She has two pieces along with a pear from her bowl of fruit and more water. On the counter there are cookies that a co-worker baked. She passes on them. She decides to leave work early because she does not have a business dinner.

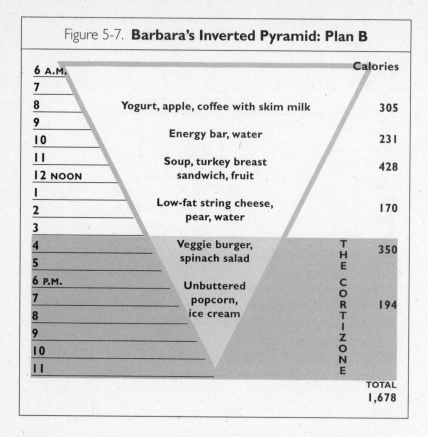

Figure 5-7. **Barbara's Inverted Pyramid: Plan B**

Time	Food	Calories
6 A.M.		Calories
7		
8	Yogurt, apple, coffee with skim milk	305
9		
10	Energy bar, water	231
11	Soup, turkey breast	428
12 NOON	sandwich, fruit	
1		
2	Low-fat string cheese, pear, water	170
3		
4	Veggie burger, spinach salad	350
5		
6 P.M.	Unbuttered popcorn, ice cream	194
7		
8		
9		
10		
11		

THE CORTIZONE

TOTAL 1,678

6:00 P.M.: Barbara heads home and prepares meat loaf and mashed potatoes for her growing children and a veggie burger and spinach salad with fruit for herself. She finishes dinner by 7:45 P.M.

8:00 P.M.: Barbara's boss calls: there's a big meeting the next morning. Barbara needs to prepare.

9:00 P.M.: The kids are doing their homework. Stressed by having to prepare for the meeting, Barbara gets the munchies while working at her computer. Before, she would have comforted herself with cookies. Now, she decides to microwave some popcorn (no butter) and eats a handful, giving the rest to the kids. Then she has a half cup of vanilla ice cream. Because she walked that afternoon, she does not feel guilty about indulging—not because she deserves it, not because she "earned" it, but because she wants it. She tastes and savors the dessert.

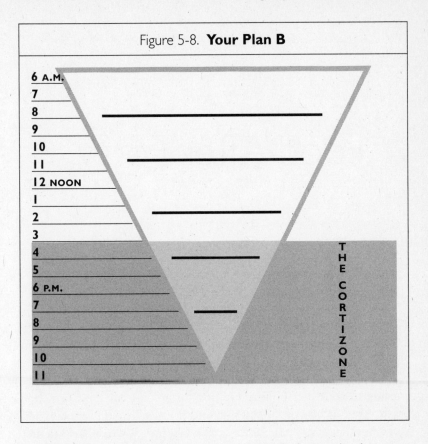

Figure 5-8. **Your Plan B**

The point is, Barbara never let any setback during the day completely destroy her commitment to High-Quality/Low-Stress foods. She allowed herself to deviate slightly without guilt or self-loathing. She looks forward to tomorrow's workout with her trainer and plans on allowing time for a forty-five-minute walk as well.

This is real life.

Next time stress hits, practice formulating your own Plan B.

Stress happens. Schedules change. People make demands on your time. The best intentions can sometimes be lost in the maze of everyday challenges and the best "diet" can hope to succeed only under optimum circumstances.

But like Barbara, as long as you plan to navigate the vulnerable times of the day, you will no longer need food and stress eating for anesthesia. Instead, you can make food work for you.

6 Food After Forty

Food is not the enemy. It never was. Now it is time to make peace with food—to understand that you must make a commitment to change your thinking about dieting and deprivation forever.

In this chapter, you will learn how to customize your eating according to your metabolism and how to prepare for the CortiZone crash. After the age of forty, it's no longer just what you eat but when you eat it that is so vital. As we saw in Chapter 5, when Barbara first came to see me, her day was exactly the opposite of what it should have been, following the stress-eating pyramid. Her whole day was scripted for disaster.

Everything changes as we turn forty. Many women in the perimenopause report that their appetite is different. As their menstrual cycles become more erratic, their female hormones begin to wax and wane unpredictably. Many women say their PMS cravings, which used to hit one to three days before the start of menses, seem to take place throughout the month.

These cravings for carbohydrates and fats (especially chocolate) may be the re-

- Determine Your Individual Energy Needs

- Eating After Forty: Dietary Requirements

- What to Eat: Protein, Carbs, Fat

sult of falling estrogen levels. Serotonin levels also decrease. If a woman's serotonin levels are low, she will have a greater interest in eating carbs to raise those levels to normal.

Another food regulator in the body is leptin, a special protein made by fat cells to signal the brain that the stomach is full. Leptin levels also decrease during the perimenopause, making women vulnerable to overeating.

Finally, at a certain critical point during perimenopause, the stress hormones plummet for eight to twelve months as estrogen levels fall. During this time, a woman feels less energetic and will desperately seek activation, most commonly through eating. Not knowing what is happening, many women become anxious about their apparent loss of control over their bodies, compounding their Toxic Stress and leading to further Toxic Weight.

As I discussed earlier, after forty our metabolism slows down. We need fewer calories to get through the day, and this means less food. So food does become more special. We need to be choosy about what we put into our bodies, especially carbohydrates and fat during the CortiZone.

Eating, however, is only part of the puzzle. No one is able to sustain a healthy life by following only one of the templates in this book. The three are codependent: developing a Stress-Resilient attitude, engaging in stress-reducing physical activity, and learning about stress-reducing eating.

In this chapter I will expand further upon the concept of Woman Food: High-Quality/Low-Stress foods that nourish and satisfy as well as fortify you against stress. I will show you the specifics of designing a Plan B for those times when everything does not go according to schedule. I will teach you how to negotiate restaurant dining as well as the importance of morning and afternoon snacks.

But we have to start at the beginning. Whenever I see a new patient, the first thing I do is determine the number of calories she needs during the day. I do this in my office with a sophisticated machine, but I can show you how to do so here with a few charts.

You need fuel to get through the day. The question is, how much? Think of calories as the units of energy you take in to fuel your body. You can get an estimate of the calories you require by doing the following calculations.

Step 1. Change your weight from pounds to kilograms by dividing your weight in pounds by 2.2.

In our example, Barbara weighs 180 pounds. Dividing this by 2.2 equals 81.8, or 82 kilograms.

Step 2. Change your height from inches to centimeters by multiplying your height in inches by 2.54.

Barbara is five feet, four inches, or 64 inches, tall. Multiplying this by 2.54 equals 162.56, or 163 centimeters.

Step 3. Use this equation to figure out the number of calories your body needs just to exist:

$$(10 \times \text{weight in kilograms}) + (6.25 \times \text{height in centimeters})$$
$$- (5 \times \text{age in years}) - 161$$

(This equation is for women only—it doesn't work for men.)
For Barbara:

$$(10 \times 82) + (6.25 \times 163) - (5 \times 41) - 161$$
$$= (820) + (1,018.75) - (205) - (161)$$
$$= 1,472.75, \text{ or } 1,473 \text{ calories}$$

So Barbara needs 1,473 calories just for her body to breathe and function at rest. In scientific terms, this is known as the "resting metabolic rate," or RMR.

Complete Work Sheet 1 to get your resting metabolic rate.

Work Sheet 1: Resting Metabolic Rate

1. What is your weight in pounds?

2. What is your weight in kilograms? To get kilograms, divide your weight in pounds by 2.2.

3. What is your height in inches?

> **4.** What is your height in centimeters? To get centimeters, multiply your height in inches by 2.54.
>
> **5.** What is your age?
>
> **6.** Insert your weight in kilograms, your height in centimeters, and your age into the following equation:
>
> 10 × your weight in kilograms + 6.25 × your height in centimeters − 5 × your age in years − 161
>
> **7.** The answer is your RMR, or resting metabolic rate.

Next we take into consideration your activity level.

Step 4. Estimate how active you are. If you have a desk job and spend your evenings in front of the computer or television, consider yourself to be sedentary or engaged in light activity. If you spend your days doing light lifting and walking, consider yourself to be in the moderate category. (As a point of reference, about 65 percent of Americans fall into the light to moderate category.) If you lift heavy objects or work with heavy machinery (in other words, you work up a sweat most of the day), consider yourself in the strenuous category. To calculate your energy (calorie) needs for the day, multiply your RMR by 1.4 if you are in the sedentary or light category, 1.6 if you are in the moderate category, or 1.9 if you're in the strenuous category.

Barbara's activity level puts her in the sedentary or light category, so we multiply her RMR by 1.4:

1,473 calories × 1.4 = 2,062.2, or 2,062 calories

Barbara therefore needs 2,062 calories to maintain her current weight of 180 pounds at her current activity level. It's important to realize that this is just an estimate, a quick rule of thumb. The calories you need in a day are also affected by your body composition, Toxic Stress level, medical status, medications you may be on, and genetics. Also, different days may have different caloric needs. While they may not increase or decrease tremendously, your caloric needs can vary from day to day, even week to week. What I am trying to do here is give you a baseline projection of your average caloric needs. Complete Work Sheet 2 to get an estimate of your caloric needs.

Barbara became a patient of mine because she was eager to lose weight. To accomplish that, she would need to take in fewer calories than her daily requirement. Experts agree that drastic reductions in calories can backfire and that a small reduction, between 250 and 500 calories per day, is more easily maintained. Let's say that Barbara decides to reduce her daily intake of calories by 250, taking in 1,812 calories for the day. (To make the calculations easier, we can round this number to 1,800.)

$$2,062 \text{ calories} - 250 = 1,800 \text{ calories}$$

At the same time, she increases her exercise to burn an additional 250 calories daily. She will thus create an "energy debt" of 500 calories a day. That's the number of calories she reduced from her diet *plus* the number of calories she expended by exercising.

Since one pound of fat weight equals 3,500 calories, she should lose about one pound of fat per week (7×500 calories = 3,500 calories) if she continues to exercise on a daily basis and keep her calories

---

Work Sheet 2: Your Caloric Needs

1. Figure out your activity level, and use the appropriate number below as a multiplier.
   a. If you are in the sedentary to light category, multiply your RMR by 1.4.
   b. If you are in the moderate category, multiply your RMR by 1.6.
   c. If you are in the strenuous category, multiply your RMR by 1.9.

RMR x activity level = calories needed to maintain your current weight

2. To lose weight, subtract up to 500 calories from your maintenance calories you calculated in step 1.

at 1,800, which is in the healthy range for her height and body composition.

More critically, Barbara reversed her eating to follow the inverted pyramid. By consuming the majority of her calories before the Corti-Zone, she was burning the "fuel" during the biologically most efficient part of her day, when her metabolism was the highest.

I know what you're thinking: "If I cut even more calories and exercise like a demon, I can lose weight faster."

First of all, health experts agree that as a general rule, you should not take in fewer than 1,200 calories a day unless you are under the supervision of a medical professional. Second, this plan is not about deprivation, and we're not into diet speak, where the fewer calories you eat and the more you sweat, the more you suffer, the better person you are. When you take in too few calories and your physical activity expectations are too high, your chances of being able to follow through with either over the long term are slim. Remember:

- **Do not go below 1,200 calories per day.**
- **Add physical activity to your daily routine to improve your fitness level and burn more calories.**

Just remember that everything I am discussing involves making the equation work for you. How do you do that? The optimal way to shed your over-forty weight is to control the amount of food you eat and the physical activity you engage in to burn that fuel (see Figure 6-1).

Not increasing your daily physical activity, whether at work or at play, and overconsuming calories will keep your daily energy expenditure equation in weight-gain mode.

Figure 6-1. **Energy Balance Equation**		
Total Energy Expenditure =	**Energy In (Food)** −	**Energy Out (Activity)**

■ Removing Weight

One day, my patient Marilyn came in for a follow-up consultation. When she had first sought my help four years before, she had been a forty-six-year-old, five-foot, four-inch tall woman who weighed almost 200 pounds. Through healthy eating and regular physical activity, she had achieved a 68-pound weight loss and maintained it for the past two years. I had a real learning experience with her that afternoon. Looking at her, I congratulated her on losing the weight and sustaining the loss for so long, which was a great triumph. Despite the diagnosis of a significant medical condition as well as the stresses of raising a family, she had minimized her usual self-destructive stress eating and had maintained her healthy lifestyle. In response to my congratulations, Marilyn sat bolt upright in her chair and stated, "Dr. Peeke, I must correct you. I did not *lose* this weight. To lose something means that you want it back, like a lost key or a lost puppy. No, Dr. Peeke, I didn't lose this weight. I *removed* it. Like garbage. I don't want it back." Marilyn's point was well taken. Her expectation of her journey with me was that she would not go back and repeat her self-destructive lifestyle; she planned to continue to live a Stress-Resilient lifestyle.

What can you expect in terms of changes in your body as you become Stress-Resilient?

If you are a woman over the age of forty, you have been weaned on quick fixes and the unrealistic expectation of instant changes in scale weight. Beware of the diet speak demons in your head. What you can achieve by eating more healthfully and exercising optimally is the continuous and sure burning of your extra fat fuel as your muscle mass gradually increases in size and calorie-burning power. Your scale weight tells you only the end result of this process. My recommendation is to step on a scale no more than every seven to ten days or, if doing so is traumatic for you, to avoid it entirely. Instead, as you begin your journey toward Stress Resilience, I would use an article of clothing as a *"clothes-o-meter"* to monitor how you, with your new fit and resilient lifestyle, feel in your clothes. For men, this may be a belt or a pair of pants. For women, it could be a jeans-o-meter or a skirt- or belt-o-meter. Try the article on once a week and watch your progress that way. If I offered you the option of a scale number weight with no guarantee of size or a very nice size but no guarantee of weight, which would you choose? Most people would opt for the size since that's what is most obvious to others. For women over the age of forty, it might be good to monitor the expanding abdomen with a tape measure, belt, or waistband, since that is where Toxic Weight lies. As your abdominal girth decreases, your risk of disease decreases as well. This is a win-win situation.

Finally, don't have unrealistic expectations of your body, dooming yourself to fail. Your Toxic Weight did not appear overnight, and it will take time to remove it. But, that's okay. Developing Stress Resilience is about being healthy, and weight removal is only one component of that. You will become healthier and feel better when you begin this journey.

■ Foods of the Future

Food provides more than calories.

It is usually the center of any celebration and, therefore, a form of entertainment and a means of pleasure. Look at some of our favorite cookbooks: *The Joy of Cooking, Mastering the Art of French Cooking.* A friend of mine stays up every night watching Emeril "take it up a notch" on the Food Network. Chefs have become the new celebrities in America.

We don't usually invite friends over to watch us mow the lawn. But we do invite them for dinner, brunch, Thanksgiving, Christmas. Thanks to the kitchen/family room combination, we now invite them over to watch us cook.

Cooking schools are overrun with applicants. Aspiring chefs and gourmands study reviews and articles like a bookie studying the pink sheet at the racetrack. What's in, what's out. New vegetable hybrids are on the market, along with the hottest trends. Risotto, not rice. Field greens. Fusion.

There's much more information now about the foods we eat and their nutritional values. We are more aware of what we eat than our mothers were. We know that food is a source of vitamins, minerals, and other nourishing gems such as phytochemicals and antioxidants. When we are in search of High-Quality/Low-Stress foods, we have to think in terms of a balance, weighing the vitamins, minerals, and other nutrients in foods against the calories those foods provide. The recommendations for a healthy dietary intake for women after forty can be seen in Figure 6-2.

Please note that in each category, we are stressing High-Quality/Low-Stress foods. Your dietary intake must include a healthy balance of protein, carbohydrate, and fat. Robust biochemical processes that support every system in your body need to be supplied with whole foods, which provide these essential nutrients.

Beware becoming "carbophobic" and leaving out all carbs. As I mentioned in the last chapter (see "Going Against the Grain"), your job is to find out which of the High-Quality/Low-Stress carbs work best for you and then include them in a healthy balance in your diet. We'll talk more about this later.

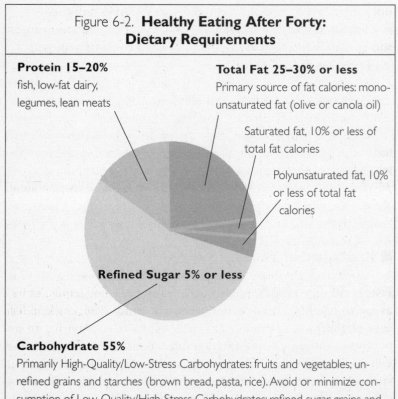

Figure 6-2. **Healthy Eating After Forty: Dietary Requirements**

Protein 15–20%
fish, low-fat dairy, legumes, lean meats

Total Fat 25–30% or less
Primary source of fat calories: mono-unsaturated fat (olive or canola oil)

Saturated fat, 10% or less of total fat calories

Polyunsaturated fat, 10% or less of total fat calories

Refined Sugar 5% or less

Carbohydrate 55%
Primarily High-Quality/Low-Stress Carbohydrates: fruits and vegetables; unrefined grains and starches (brown bread, pasta, rice). Avoid or minimize consumption of Low-Quality/High-Stress Carbohydrates: refined sugar, grains and starches.

■ A Protein Primer

We get calories from the protein, fats, and carbohydrates in our foods. Every gram of protein or carbohydrate we consume supplies four calories. Every gram of fat we consume supplies nine calories, which means that fat supplies more than twice as many calories as protein or carbohydrates. So for women over forty, protein is a critical energy source that is also relatively low in calories.

Protein is needed for the growth and repair of body tissues such as muscles, blood, bones, hair, skin, and nails. Hormones and infection-fighting antibodies are also proteins. Research shows that protein requirements may actually increase as you age, to about .4 to .5 gram of protein per pound of body weight. The reason is not entirely clear, but it could be based on metabolism: the midlife female body does not use protein as efficiently as it did a couple of decades ago.

The good news? You can easily reach your protein needs by ensuring that about 20 percent of your calories come from protein.

In Barbara's case:

$$0.20 \times 1,800 = 360$$

That means 360 calories from various protein sources. Since protein has 4 calories per gram, to figure out the number of grams of protein Barbara should consume daily, we divide the protein calories by 4: $360 \div 4 = 90$ grams of protein. What does this mean in terms of food?

■ Protein Sources

Fish, shellfish, mollusks, poultry, dry beans, peas, and lentils, as well as egg whites, are terrific protein providers. In addition, chicken, fish, eggs, soybeans, and peanuts are rich sources of vitamin B_6, an important nutrient for women during this time of life. Because our metabolism is changing, our need for vitamin B_6 is increasing. Also, vitamin B_6 is necessary to produce serotonin, and when serotonin levels are normal, we have less craving for carbohydrate and sweets. Adequate vitamin B_6 may be needed to avert stress. Vitamin B_6 is necessary for the development and maintenance of the nervous system, which includes adrenaline production. Even a small deficiency of vitamin B_6 is associated with mood disturbances, such as depression, anxiety, and lack of energy. Therefore, it is essential to maintain adequate levels of vitamin B_6 in the diet.

Beans and Nuts

Cooked dry beans and peas are packed with protein. These low-fat protein sources are also loaded with dietary fiber. In addition, soybeans and soy-based products such as soy milk and tofu are rich sources of phytoestrogens, weak estrogens found in plants. These seem to act in a woman's body in two ways: They bind to estrogen receptors and block them so that the body's natural estrogens can't bind at those sites. They also appear to reduce the amount of biologically active estrogen, which as you now know can encourage fat storage in perimenopausal women.

Soy products include

- **Fresh soybeans**
- **Canned or frozen soybeans**
- **Dried raw soybeans**
- **Soy nuts**
- **Soy milk**
- **Tofu**
- **Tempeh**
- **Miso**
- **Soy flour**
- **Soy protein powders**
- **Soy butter**
- **Soy breakfast cereals**
- **Soy burgers and hot dogs**
- **Soy energy bars**

Other sources of phytoestrogens are

- **Chickpeas**
- **Lentils**
- **Clover**
- **Onions**

■ **Apples**
■ **Red wine**

In premenopausal women, phytoestrogens protect against breast cancer. In perimenopausal women, who have lower estrogen levels than premenopausal women, phytoestrogens protect not only the breasts but also the heart and bones. Furthermore, according to studies of menopausal women conducted in Asian countries, where women's diets are high in phytoestrogens, hot flashes are not as prevalent as they are in America.

Another good protein source is peanut butter. This is higher in fat than fish, poultry, and beans, but the major type of fat in peanut butter is monounsaturated, or "good," fat.

Lean Red Meats

Lean red meats are higher in saturated fat than other protein sources, so it's best not to rely on them to fulfill your protein needs. I'm not going to tell anyone to give up red meat, but some of my patients have made that choice and are happy with the results.

The best red meat choices should be well trimmed, even lean cuts of beef such as flank, sirloin, tenderloin, round, T-bone, or porterhouse steak. Other good choices are cubed, round, rib, or chuck steak, rump roast, and ground beef that is labeled "90 percent lean."

Pork is a good source of protein, and the cuts available at the grocery store seem to be getting leaner. Pork tenderloins often come premarinated. Other healthy pork products are well-trimmed cuts like fresh, canned, cured or boiled ham, Canadian bacon, loin chops and roasts and rib chops and roasts.

Lean cuts of lamb and veal include well-trimmed cuts such as lamb roast, chops, or legs and veal chops, cutlets, and roasts.

Dairy Products

Dairy products like skim milk, nonfat yogurt and reduced-fat cheeses are also good protein providers. High-Quality/Low-Stress protein sources are lower in fat, cholesterol, and sugar compared to Low-Quality/High-Stress protein sources. Check Table 6-1 to see the foods in the different categories. Dairy products can be served as a condiment, side dish, or entree.

Dairy Tips

- ■ **Use flavored nonfat yogurt as a fruit dip.**
- ■ **Top a baked potato with herb-seasoned plain yogurt or low-fat cottage cheese.**
- ■ **Enjoy a reduced-fat cheese and vegetable pita pocket for lunch or dinner.**

In addition to protein, dairy foods provide us with calcium, a critical mineral, especially for women. Calcium is important for bone formation and maintenance. At any adult age, women have lower bone mass and density than men. It's not fair, but men have a 20 percent higher bone density than women and suffer only half the rate of bone loss over a lifetime. This translates into a 20 to 30 percent loss of bone in men compared to a 50 percent loss in women.

Everyone loses bone with age, but whether or not that loss spells the disabling condition of osteoporosis (a thinning of the bones, making them more likely to fracture) depends on how much bone we have to begin with and how quickly we lose it. Bone is always in a state of remodeling, or breaking down and building up again. At menopause, the decline in estrogen causes more bone breakdown and less bone buildup. The result? Less and weaker bone.

What about a cold glass of milk? Most of the milk in this country is fortified with vitamin D. This is great news for women, because as we age, the body has a harder time making the active form of vitamin D that ensures adequate absorption of calcium. Vitamin D also regulates the amount of calcium in our bodies. The result of an inadequate intake of vitamin D is bone softening and fractures.

Can't eat dairy? Here's how to get the calcium you need. If you can't tolerate dairy sources of calcium, you can find foods that have calcium added to them, such as some brands of soy milk, apple, orange, and grape juices and breakfast cereals. Just check the ingredient panel on the food to see if calcium has been added. Then look at the Nutrition Facts panel (see page 141 for an example) to see the percentage of the recommended daily allowance of calcium in the food.

Many of my patients take calcium supplements. Absorption of calcium supplements is best at individual doses of 500 milligrams or less, and I think calcium is best taken between meals. Women over fifty years actually need more than the daily value used for labeling, or 1,200 milligrams.

Nutrition Facts

Serving Size: 1 drink box
Amount Per Serving Calories: 120

Contains filtered water, concentrated orange juice, tricalcium phosphate and calcium lactate (calcium sources).

	% Daily Value*
Total Fat 0g	0%
Sodium 25mg	1%
Potassium 500mg	14%
Total Carbohydrate 28g	9%
Sugars 25g	
Protein 0g	
Vitamin C	130%
Calcium 150mg	15%
Thiamin	10%
Folate	15%

(Not a significant source of calories from fat, saturated fat, cholesterol, dietary fiber, vitamin A and Iron. *Percent Daily Values are based on a 2,000 calorie diet.)

■ How Much Protein Do You Need?

You'll need about five to seven ounces of meat, fish, or poultry daily. One egg, one-half cup cooked dry beans or peas, or two tablespoons of peanut butter count as one ounce of meat. You should consume about two servings of milk or other dairy foods daily. One serving is one cup of skim milk or nonfat yogurt or one and a half ounces of reduced-fat cheese.

Table 6-1. **Protein Sources**

High-Quality/Low-Stress

Chicken breast

Dry beans or peas: soybeans, black beans, kidney beans, navy beans, pinto beans, white beans, lentils, chickpeas

Egg whites

Fish: sole, haddock, fresh tuna, trout, salmon, perch, bluefish, etc.

Shellfish and mollusks: shrimp, oysters, clams, scallops, mussels, lobster

Tofu

Tuna, canned in water

Turkey or chicken breast

Reduced-fat cheeses

Nonfat yogurt

Skim milk, 1 percent milk, nonfat dry milk

Low-Quality/High-Stress

Fried chicken or, for that matter, fried anything: chicken nuggets

Heavily marbled or untrimmed red meats (high in saturated fat)

More than 4 egg yolks a week (high in cholesterol)

Breaded frozen fish, fish sticks

Cold cuts, spareribs, sausage, bacon, full-fat hot dogs

Liver

Poultry with the skin on it

Dark meat of poultry (leg, wing, thigh)

Full-fat cheeses

Low-fat flavored yogurt (it's high in sugar)

Whole milk

■ Protein Points

- ■ Fish and shellfish are lower in fat than other animal protein sources. People have been wary of including shellfish in the diets because of the cholesterol content. Here's the real story: shellfish, such as crab, scallops, mussels, and clams, have a slightly higher cholesterol content than chicken or beef. Shrimp has almost twice the cholesterol as meat. The good news is that even with the higher cholesterol content, the saturated fat content is much lower, making shellfish a nutritional bargain.

- ■ Surimi is made from Alaskan pollack, a deep-sea whitefish. The fish undergoes extensive processing before it is shaped into "crab" legs, "shrimp," or "scallops." The processing involves removing the skin and bones, grinding, washing, straining, and cooking. Sugar, salt, and other flavors and binders are often added. There are better protein sources.

- ■ The white meat of poultry has less fat than dark meat. A large amount of the fat in poultry is located in the skin. There is no need to remove the skin before cooking the poultry, but be sure to take it off before eating.

- ■ Trim the visible fat from meat to cut the fat content.

- ■ Stick to four egg yolks a week to keep a lid on your cholesterol intake.

- ■ Try a meal using cooked dry beans and peas as a protein source; beans and peas provide us with more than protein. If you're short on time, use canned beans. Just be sure to drain them and rinse them well to reduce the added sodium.

■ The Skinny on Fat

Fat is an essential part of your diet. Any woman who tries to cut all fat from her diet is on the road to disaster. Fats supply a concentrated source of energy. Some vitamins need fat to transport them in and through your body. Fat is essential for the growth and maintenance of many tissues, including the skin and nerves.

Fats can be broken down into two classes: saturated and unsaturated. Saturated fat is found in higher amounts in foods of animal origin, such as dairy products, meats, and poultry. Plant sources that are high in "sat fat" include coconut and palm oils.

Saturated fats tend to increase LDL cholesterol, often referred to as "bad" cholesterol because high levels in the blood are associated with an increased risk of heart disease.

Unsaturated fats are usually liquid at room temperature. They are found in higher amounts in plant foods. There are two types of unsaturated fats, monounsaturated and polyunsaturated. When these are substituted for saturated fats in the diet, they lower total cholesterol and LDL cholesterol.

Epidemiological evidence from Mediterranean countries suggests a possible heart-protective role for monounsaturated fats. In these countries, where people consume high levels of monounsaturates, there is a lower incidence of heart disease. Examples of foods high in monounsaturated fats include olives and olive oil, peanuts, peanut butter and peanut oil, and canola oil.

Polyunsaturated fats lower total cholesterol and LDL cholesterol. Polyunsaturated fat sources include vegetable oils such as corn, soybean, safflower, and sunflower oils. They also include the heart-protecting omega-3 fatty acids found in plentiful supply in fish such as salmon, mackerel, and tuna.

It's not smart to overdo it on the types of polyunsaturated fats that occur in vegetable oils; in animal studies, they have been linked with promotion of tumor development and suppression of the immune system.

Health experts agree that 20 to 25 percent of total calories should come from fat. Use 80 percent as your threshold.

In Barbara's case: $0.20–0.25 \times 1,800 = 360–450$ calories should come from fat. Fat has 9 calories per gram, so to determine the number of grams of fat Barbara should eat daily, we just divide the fat calories by 9: $360 \div 9 = 40$ grams, $450 \div 9 = 50$ grams, making her fat range 40 to 50 grams daily.

Fat has both positives and negatives. On the plus side, it gives food flavor, improves the texture of many foods, and is satisfying. On the down side, it is calorie dense, so foods high in fat are also usually high in calories. When planning your fat intake, minimize saturated fat, go easy on the polyunsaturated vegetable oils, and make up the bulk of your fat intake with monounsaturated fat and sources of omega-3 fatty acids.

In percentages, this means that no more than 7 percent of fat intake should come from saturated fat, no more than 10 percent should come from polyunsaturated fat, and the remaining (and greatest) percentage should come from monounsaturated fat.

What does this mean in terms of food? Fat becomes part of your diet in three ways:

1. **Some foods, such as oils, salad dressings, cream, butter, and margarine, are obviously mostly fat. Use these foods sparingly and focus on reducing saturated and replacing it with monounsaturated sources.**

2. **Foods that come from animals (such as meat, fish, poultry, eggs, milk, yogurt, and cheese) are generally naturally higher in fat than foods that come from plants. However, there are many nonfat, low-fat, and lean choices available—take advantage of them! Refer to Table 6-1 and choose the High-Quality/Low-Stress Foods whenever possible.**

3. **Fat can enter the diet through food preparation. Frying adds unnecessary fat and calories to perfectly innocent**

Table 6-2. **Fried Foods**

Food	Amount	Calories When Not Fried	Calories When Fried (in 6± T oil)
Cauliflower	130 g (about 4½ oz)	25	250
Chicken	1 breast	142	218
Egg	1	77	91
Onions	105 g (about ½ cup)	46	262
Potatoes	78 g (about ½ cup)	68	246
Shrimp	2 oz	88	137

foods, as you can see in Table 6-2. Try grilling, broiling, boil-
ing, poaching, baking, and roasting. Pass up cream sauces or
greatly reduce your use of them.

■ Freedom from Fat-Free Foods

If less fat is good, is no fat better? Unfortunately, many women have
learned the hard way that the answer to this is no.

Nutritionists used to say that to lose weight, you should just eat
less fat. Then food manufacturers began to develop fat-free foods:
salad dressings, cookies, ice cream, sour cream, and so on. Unfortunately, the fat was replaced with a large amount of sugar, so the calorie savings evaporated.

Also, these guiltless goodies are easy to gulp and overconsume
rather than taste and savor. I have stopped counting the number of
my patients who love fat-free cookies so much they eat a whole
box—at one sitting.

Fat-free foods also introduced women to foods they had never
eaten before, so instead of reducing the calories in their diet, they actually added calories. Barbara never ate cream cheese on a regular
basis until fat-free cream cheese came out. Then she had it every
morning. She also ate cookies once in a while, but when fat-free cookies became available, she ate some every night. Because they were fat-
free, she ate a few more. By consuming fat-free foods to excess,
Barbara added extra calories in her diet that weren't there before.

Check the ingredient lists and the Nutrition Facts of fat-free
foods. See how many calories there are in a serving. Use the products
wisely. If they're lower-fat, lower-calorie versions of what you usually have, consider them a bargain. If you never or rarely eat the full-
fat version, pass on the reduced-fat or fat-free version. Think of
fat-free foods as "sale" items: just because they're on sale doesn't
mean we need, want, or have to buy them.

■ Carbs: The Constant Craving

Carbohydrate-rich foods are energy sources; in fact, the body prefers
to use carbs as fuel. Foods that are high in carbohydrates can be excellent fiber sources if chosen wisely.

The recommended amount of carbohydrate in our diets ranges

from 55 to 60 percent of our daily caloric intake. In Barbara's case, this means that the total amount of carbohydrate would be

$$1,800 \times 55–60\% = 990–1,080 \text{ calories}$$

Since carbohydrate has 4 calories per gram, this amounts to 248 to 270 grams of total carbohydrate.

Carbohydrates are found primarily in grains, fruits, and vegetables. Protein foods that contain carbohydrates are milk and yogurt, as well as dried beans, peas, and lentils. Carbohydrates have taken some hard knocks during the past few years. I believe that most of the problem has to do with some misconceptions about them.

The Carb Clock

All carbohydrates are not created equal. Different sources of carbohydrates have their own unique effects on insulin and blood sugar. Some carbohydrates (such as sugar-coated cornflakes) produce an immediate and dramatic rise in blood sugar, resulting in very high levels of insulin. As you recall, insulin is one of the most potent stimulants to appetite. It is important to keep insulin levels low enough not to stimulate excess appetite.

Through trial and error, you will discover your own insulin sensitivity to foods that contain carbohydrate. Foods that tend to drive up your appetite should be minimized or avoided. You can learn to live without Count Chocula cereal!

To decrease the chance that carbs will drive up appetite, especially under stress, it is important to remember that it's not just the *quality* and the *quantity* of the carbohydrates ingested, but what *time* you are eating your carbs! I have devised a Carb Clock to help you remember when to eat which carbs. The key is to remember that:

- ✔ **The cutoff time is about 5 P.M.**
- ✔ **Fruits and vegetables may be eaten before and after 5 P.M.**
- ✔ **High-Quality/Low-Stress carbs from grains should be eaten primarily before 5 P.M. and should generally not be included for dinner, except perhaps once per week**
- ✔ **Low-Quality/High-Stress carbs should be avoided or minimized at all times**

After the age of forty, it is imperative that women realize that carbohydrate ingestion involves some real thought. We no longer need the intense carb fueling we used to need when we played field hockey or spent half the afternoon jumping rope. We are metabolically different, and we must embrace eating behavior more appropriate for our age and gender.

The Glycemic Index

Food scientists have developed a ranking system of foods based upon their effect on blood sugar and therefore insulin. This is called the glycemic index, and it is helpful to know which foods to watch out for and which foods you can safely eat without significantly boosting your blood sugar. Remember, what works for you may be different for the next woman. The foods on the glycemic index are compared to a standard, usually glucose or white bread, that has a value of 100. See Table 6-3 for the glycemic indexes of common foods.

Foods are considered to have a high glycemic index if they have a value above 70. Foods with a low glycemic index have values less than 55. All others elevate blood sugar levels moderately.

Foods should never be rated as "good" or "bad" based on their

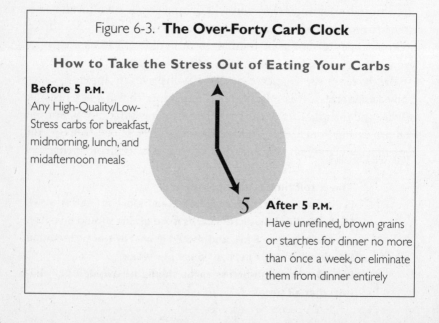

Figure 6-3. **The Over-Forty Carb Clock**

How to Take the Stress Out of Eating Your Carbs

Before 5 P.M.
Any High-Quality/Low-Stress carbs for breakfast, midmorning, lunch, and midafternoon meals

After 5 P.M.
Have unrefined, brown grains or starches for dinner no more than once a week, or eliminate them from dinner entirely

Table 6-3. **Glycemic Index of Common Sources of Carbohydrates**

Food	Glycemic Index (based on white bread)
Bakery Products/Breads	
Bagel, white	103
Bread, white	100
Bread, oat bran	68
Bread, pumpernickel	58
Bread, mixed grain	64
Croissant	96
Doughnut	108
Hamburger bun	87
Melba toast	100
Muffins (commercial)	84–98
Waffle	109
Cereals	
All bran	43
Cheerios	106
Corn flakes	110
Grape Nuts	96
Oatmeal (one-minute)	93
Puffed wheat	96
Rice Krispies	117
Shredded Wheat	96
Total	109
Cookies/Crackers	
Oatmeal cookies	77
Vanilla wafers	110
Rice cakes	117
Fruit/Fruit Juice (Unsweetened)	
Apple	52
Apple juice	58
Apricots, dried	44

Banana	76
Grapefruit	36
Grapefruit juice	69
Grapes	62
Orange	62
Orange juice	74
Pear	51
Raisins	91

Grains

Rice, brown	79
Rice, white	81

Milk/Milk Products

Ice cream, low-fat	71
Milk, skim	46
Yogurt, low-fat	47

Legumes

Beans, dried and cooked	40
Chickpeas	47
Lentils	41
Peanuts	21
Soybeans	25

Pasta

Spaghetti, white	59

Sugars

Fructose	32
Sucrose	92

Vegetables

Carrots	101
Corn	78
Peas, green	68
Potato, white	80
Potato, sweet	77

Sources: K. Foster-Powell and J. B. Miller (1995), "International tables of glycemic index," *American Journal of Clinical Nutrition* 62(4):871S–890S; J. Brand-Miller and K. Foster-Powell (1999), "Diets with a low glycemic index: from theory to practice," *Nutrition Today* 34(2):64–72.

glycemic index. Instead, just consider their balance in the diet. Don't avoid foods with a high glycemic index altogether; instead, try to balance the foods you eat. Try to eat a low-glycemic-index food at each meal. For example, at breakfast, you may want to have a bowl of cereal (high glycemic index) with skim milk (low glycemic index) and one-half grapefruit (low glycemic index), rather than just grabbing a bagel and coffee.

MYTH: All carbohydrates are alike.
FACT: There are High-Quality/Low-Stress carbohydrates and Low-Quality/High-Stress carbohydrates (see Table 6-5). High-Quality/Low-Stress carbohydrates are foods that give you more than calories. They provide dietary fiber and some essential vitamins and minerals. Whole grain breads and cereals, brown rice, whole wheat pasta, dried peas, beans, and lentils, skim, 1 percent, and nonfat dry milk, nonfat yogurt, and fruits and vegetables fall into this category.

In addition to being sources of dietary fiber, fruits and vegetables are gold mines when it comes to vitamins (especially vitamin C), minerals, and phytochemicals.

Vitamin C appears to be intimately involved in the stress response. Animal and human studies have shown that it may be used to detoxify chemicals that are released during stress, and that it may be required for an adequate response to a stressful situation. Citrus fruits, strawberries, kiwifruit, peppers, cabbage, and broccoli are examples of fruits and vegetables packed with vitamin C.

Phytochemicals are compounds found in fruits and vegetables that have many beneficial effects. They appear to halt cancer at every stage of its development. For example, chemicals in tomatoes block the formation of cancer-causing substances; chemicals in broccoli push the cancer-promoting agent out of the cell; chemicals in cabbage work at the enzyme level to prevent cell mutations.

Fruits and vegetables also add flavor, color, and texture to your meals. The best way to eat more of them is to make sure they're ready to eat so that you don't have to think about peeling, slicing, or dicing them when you want something fast. Also, don't relegate them just to meals—use them for snacking too.

Fiber Facts

Whole fruits and vegetables have more fiber than juices; experiment with different fruits to find the ones that satisfy you; steer clear of sauces or dips for fruits and vegetables, as these can add extra fat and calories.

Fiber is the structural part of plant foods that can't be digested by enzymes in our intestines. Fiber has special benefits. It helps prevent and treat constipation, which is a common complaint among perimenopausal women. It may also prevent some types of cancer, particularly colon cancer.

Fiber can help stabilize blood sugar levels by slowing the absorption of sugars (glucose) in foods. Studies have also shown that fiber lowers blood cholesterol levels. Most women consume only about half of the recommended range of 20 to 35 grams of fiber daily. Good fiber sources are wheat bran, corn bran, oat bran, most bran breakfast cereals, oatmeal, whole wheat fiber products, cooked dry beans, peas, and lentils, and most fruits and vegetables.

Low-Quality/High-Stress carbohydrates include foods that lack substantial dietary fiber and those that are or contain an abundance of added sugars. Sugars include white sugar, brown sugar, raw sugar, corn syrup, honey, and molasses. These foods give energy, but not much else in the way of nutrition. Added sugars can be found in foods such as candy and soft drinks, jams, jellies, and sugars added

Table 6-4. **Added Sugars in Common Foods**

Food	Amount	Added Sugar (in teaspoons)
Doughnut	1 medium	2
Cake, frosted	1/16 of average size	6
Pie, fruit, 2 crusts	1/6 of an 8-inch pie	6
Fruit, canned in heavy syrup	1/2 cup	4
Low-fat yogurt, fruit	8 oz	7
Chocolate shake	10 fluid oz	9
Cola	12 fluid oz	9
Fruit drink	12 fluid oz	12

Source: "The Food Guide Pyramid," *Home and Garden Bulletin* 252, USDA, 1998.

at the table. For a real eye-opener, look at Table 6-4 to see the number of teaspoons of added sugars in some common foods.

I recommend that no more than 10 percent of the carbohydrate calories come from simple sugars. In Barbara's case, this means: .10 × (990–1,080) = 99–108 calories from added simple sugars. Since sugar has 16 calories per teaspoon, this means that Barbara should have no more than 6 to 7 teaspoons of added sugar daily.

MYTH: "Because many carbohydrate foods are low in fat, I can eat as much as I want."

FACT: While it is true that many carbohydrate sources are low in fat, they still provide calories. Eating more calories than you need of any food results in extra weight. Portion size is the key when it comes to carbohydrate. For example, a one-ounce bagel is one serving. We haven't seen a one-ounce bagel in years—most of the bagels you buy are three to four times that weight. Another example is rice or pasta. A portion of rice or pasta is one-half cup cooked. When we eat at a restaurant, we are usually served a mountain of pasta—often two to three cups. We struggle mightily, but we end up eating most of it "because it's there."

Portions of this size can cause bloating, because when carbohydrate is stored in the body, it stores water along with it. You might notice that if you overdo certain carbohydrates (such as bread, pasta, noodles, or rice) at the evening meal or later in the night, you retain fluid or feel bloated the next morning. Physically, this is not a problem. The fluid is not body fat. Psychologically, it could be a disaster. We have found that when women start the day feeling defeated, their control is at an all-time low.

If you aren't satisfied with a small serving of these types of carbohydrate foods at dinner and you notice a fluid retention problem, enjoy the foods at lunch and avoid them at the evening meal.

MYTH: "I can lose weight really quickly if I really restrict the carbohydrate I eat."

FACT: Our bodies prefer to use carbohydrate as fuel. We should eat at least 6 servings daily from the grain group, 5 to 6 servings from the fruit group, and 6 to 8 servings from the vegetable group. If we severely restrict the carbohydrates in our diets, we will lose

---

Table 6-5. **Carbohydrate Sources**

High-Quality/Low-Stress
Whole grain breads
Whole grain cereals
Brown rice
Whole wheat pasta
Skim, 1%, or nonfat dry milk
Biscuits
Dried cooked beans, peas, lentils
Vegetables and fruits

Low-Quality/High-Stress
White bread
Sweetened cereals
White rice
White pasta
Nonfat yogurt
Croissants
Doughnuts
Cakes and sugars

---

weight, but it will be fluid, or "water weight," not fat weight. Fat weight is the Toxic Weight. Diets that prescribe limited amounts of carbohydrate are not well balanced.

Now that you know *what* to eat, you need to understand *when* to eat. After the age of forty, you must eat according to the CortiZone. This means eating every three hours. As we have already seen, your eating should be like an inverted pyramid. Fuel up in the morning by eating breakfast. Make sure you eat a satisfying lunch. Taper down your eating as evening approaches. As a rule of thumb, consume about 60 to 65 percent of your calories before you sit down to dinner.

For example, because Barbara's daily intake is 1,800 calories, she should try to consume 1,080 to 1,170 calories by 5 or 6 P.M. Have planned snacks, especially at the times when your cortisol levels are low. Make sure your meals and snacks are balanced in protein, carbohydrates, and fat.

■ Get to Know Your H₂O

For women over forty, the importance of water cannot be overstated. Water has so many functions in the body: It acts as a solvent for nutrients and waste products in the body; it transports nutrients to cells; it regulates temperature; it lubricates the joints; and it provides moisture to the skin. Lower estrogen levels during perimenopause make water intake even more critical. Women will notice that their skin is drier at this time of life. They may also be plagued with more urinary tract infections due to the changes in their hormones.

Strive to drink eight glasses of water daily. Plain water, seltzer, and mineral water are all good choices. Watch out for beverages that increase fluid loss from the body. Alcohol and caffeinated beverages (coffee, tea, colas) are the main culprits.

■ The Cocktail Hour

While moderate amounts of wine have been linked with lowering the risk of heart disease, the negatives of alcohol consumption are food for thought. Think about the following facts.

- Alcohol has seven calories per gram, almost as many as fat. Mixers add even more calories.
- Research has shown that alcohol may be toxic to bones. A marked reduction in bone remodeling occurs when alcohol is consumed. Although alcoholics are at greatest risk, even moderate alcohol (6 ounces per day) intake has been associated with an increased risk of hip and forearm fractures.
- Alcohol reduces control, which can result in choosing foods that are high in fat and calories.

■ The Lowdown on Double Lattes

Women love coffee. We take it black, with cream and sugar, with cinnamon and frothy milk. Decaf, double decaf. There seems to be an upscale coffee bar on every corner. We rely on caffeine to give us a boost when our energy levels are low. Caffeine is found in coffee, tea, colas, chocolate, and some over-the-counter medications.

Caffeine can have a negative effect on bone. Researchers have found that women who drink at least two cups of caffeinated coffee daily have lower bone densities than those who did not. There is some good news, however. The effects of caffeine are offset in women who drink at least one glass of milk daily. The bottom line is this: if you are going to drink caffeinated beverages, limit the amount and include milk in your diet daily.

Caffeine can also make you more sensitive to changes in your blood sugar. If this happens in the late afternoon, when you're in the CortiZone, chances are you'll head for the nearest vending machine to soothe the dizziness and shakes. And contrary to those wistful gourmet coffee commercials, caffeine does absolutely nothing to alleviate stress.

■ Making It All Work

By now you are aware that you can help to curb your stress eating by sticking to foods that don't overly stress the body. These High-Quality/Low-Stress foods are your ticket to maintaining greater resilience in the face of daily events that would normally send you to the vending machine. Learning to navigate the CortiZone with these foods and planning ahead of time to eat well during this vulnerable time of day is about 80 percent of the battle. Finally, remember that your dietary intake requires a balance of foods. Try to plan your fats, carbs, and proteins for the day with that in mind. Keep your Carb Clock in mind as a daily reminder of what to eat and when.

In the next chapter, we'll apply these principles to real time stresses and learn how to avoid stress eating through regrouping and continually practicing resilient eating habits.

7 Fight Fat Right

■ Eating and Regrouping

The key to destressing the eating process is learning how to regroup when your basic routine has been interrupted by daily life events. Deb's story can teach you some of the essentials.

Deb came to me almost two years ago complaining of crushing fatigue. A lifelong stress eater, five feet, nine inches tall, and large-boned, Deb, at forty-three, was a successful but stressed computer expert who was beginning to show high blood pressure. Obesity, diabetes, and heart disease ran in her father's side of the family. As she was entering menopause, for the first time in her life she was deeply worried that she would develop these health problems. As she stood on the scale, I watched the number climb to 250 pounds.

■ Plan A and Plan B: How to Eat When You Can't Eat According to Plan

■ Portion Control

■ Menus for Your Stress Profile

■ Destressing Perimenopause with Food

We began to work together. After one year, she lost 50 pounds while her husband, who was extremely supportive, lost 25 pounds. Together, they worked out and began to live more healthfully.

How did she do it?

Like Barbara, she adopted the Stress-Eating Inverted Pyramid model (see page 160) and made the commitment to prioritize the earlier part of the day for her consumption of healthy food. A classic Stress Overeater, she had been having most of her calories during the CortiZone. We worked together to reprogram her meal planning.

To see what Deb was doing wrong and how we corrected it, refer to Table 7-1 and Figures 7-1 and 7-2.

Just to maintain her weight of 250 pounds, Deb would have to consume approximately 2,000 to 2,500 calories per day. Her goal, of course, was to remove her Toxic Weight. Her newly revised routine, or Plan A, now includes a caloric intake of 1,500 to 1,800 calories per day with a much higher level of physical activity.

Deb learned to practice one of my cardinal principles for de-stressing the eating process: **BYOF: Bring Your Own Food.**

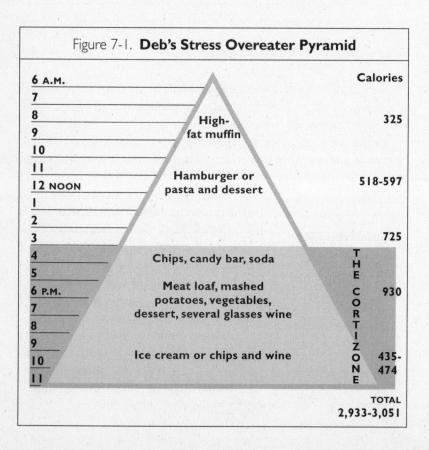

Figure 7-1. **Deb's Stress Overeater Pyramid**

Time	Food		Calories
6 A.M.			Calories
7			
8	High-fat muffin		325
9			
10			
11			
12 NOON	Hamburger or pasta and dessert		518-597
1			
2			
3			725
4	Chips, candy bar, soda	T H E	
5			
6 P.M.	Meat loaf, mashed potatoes, vegetables, dessert, several glasses wine	C O R T I Z O N E	930
7			
8			
9			
10	Ice cream or chips and wine		435-474
11			

TOTAL
2,933-3,051

Table 7-1. **Deb's Eating Plans, Before and After**

Before: Old Plan A	After: New Plan A
Food	
Breakfast	
High-fat muffin	Cereal, skim milk, fruit
Midmorning Snack	
None	Fruit, yogurt, water
Lunch	
Large restaurant meal: hamburger, pasta, or steak-and-cheese sandwich with dessert	Turkey sandwich full of salad greens and tomato from home, bag of baby carrots, fruit, water
Midafternoon Snack	
Vending machine or cafeteria at work: chips, pretzels, candy bar, office kitchen snacks, sodas	Low-fat string cheese, yogurt, cottage cheese, crackers or cup of soup, and fruit
Dinner	
Large restaurant portions of pasta, meat loaf, or fried chicken, with mashed potatoes or veggies and dessert, as well as several glasses of wine. Usually after 8 P.M.	Primarily home eating: salad, veggies, fruit, and protein source such as fish, veggie burger, chicken. Occasional glass of wine. By 8 P.M.
After-Dinner Snack	
Cookies, ice cream, chips, wine	Occasional fruit or popcorn
Exercise	
None	Walks three miles per day with husband and lifts weights twice per week with trainer
Dress Size	
20	14

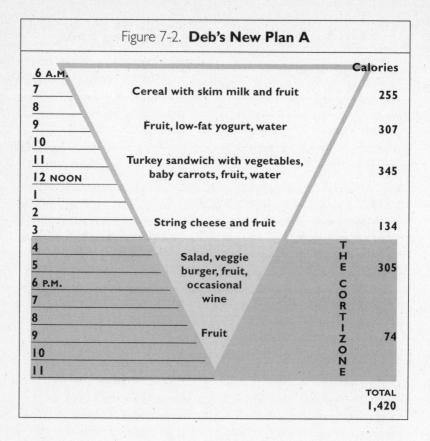

Figure 7-2. **Deb's New Plan A**

Time	Food	Calories
6 A.M.		
7	Cereal with skim milk and fruit	255
8		
9	Fruit, low-fat yogurt, water	307
10		
11	Turkey sandwich with vegetables, baby carrots, fruit, water	345
12 NOON		
1		
2		
3	String cheese and fruit	134
4		
5	Salad, veggie burger, fruit, occasional wine	305
6 P.M.		
7		
8		
9	Fruit	74
10		
11		

THE CORTIZONE

TOTAL 1,420

When you plan and are prepared with food throughout your busy day, whether you are traveling, at the office, or in your car, you will always be able to feed yourself despite life stresses that might interfere with your Plan A meals. In essence, you are constantly prepared for Plan B, which is a modified Plan A, revised to adapt to a life stress. Let's look at an example in Deb's life.

After one year, Deb had removed more than 50 pounds of excess fat weight and had increased her fitness level significantly. About that time, she walked into my office for one of her follow-up appointments and, smiling, handed me a Polaroid picture. I gasped. The snapshot showed a huge oak tree that, during a severe thunder storm two weeks earlier, had been hit by lightning. The tree had toppled over onto her lovely two-story Colonial home, obliterating her bedroom and half of the second floor. Fortunately, she and her family hadn't been home at the time and no one had been hurt.

"Before I met you," Deb said, "I would have eaten a mountain of food over this crisis. For that matter, I would have stepped into my refrigerator and just lived there. But instead I just stood in the street with my husband as we realized that "It's life," and we would be okay.

Deb had learned to regroup by stepping back and seeing that this life stress was not worth self-destructing over. I congratulated her and talked with her about how she was going to realistically work around this crisis. Deb stated that it would be wise for her to take some time to deal with the crisis as a priority while simply maintaining her current weight of 198 pounds, a 52-pound weight loss thus far. She was practicing another destressing principle:

When a significant stress hits your life, learn to "tread weight," and do not self-destruct.

For the next ten months, Deb continued to maintain her weight well as she went about the tedious work of dealing with insurance agents and rebuilding her home. Then she regrouped and felt she was ready to continue to shed more excess fat and put more time and effort into her exercise routine. It is important to note that one of Deb's greatest accomplishments was the ability to maintain her new body composition and fitness levels for almost a year while dealing with the house and her daily life stresses. Deb has much to be proud about. She had mastered Stress Resilience through her regrouping efforts.

We must all develop a Plan A for those times when life is going smoothly and according to schedule. Unexpected events happen infrequently, so that most of the time we can follow it.

The following are the Golden Rules of Plan A:

■ **At each main meal, remember to include about 55 percent carbohydrates, prioritizing complex carbs, 15–20 percent protein, and approximately 25–30 percent fat.**
■ **If you eat breakfast before 7 A.M., your snack three hours later should include a protein source (e.g., yogurt) as well**

as fruit, assuming you eat lunch between 12 and 1 P.M. If you eat breakfast after 8 A.M., your midmorning snack should be just a piece of fruit.

■ You should have your midafternoon snack three hours after you eat lunch. This snack should definitely include protein as well as carbohydrates and minimal amounts of fat. Examples: soup with crackers, low-fat or fat-free cottage cheese with fruit, yogurt and fruit, or low-fat string cheese and fruit.

■ Avoid consuming the majority of your calories during the CortiZone. Consume most (65 percent) of your total calories for the day before dinner (by 5 P.M.).

■ Watch your timing! If you eat after 8 P.M., you'll gain weight.

■ Destress eating during the CortiZone by having an eating plan to rely on.

■ Be prepared to make the transition to Plan B when significant stress occurs.

■ Don't skip meals.

■ Drink eight eight-ounce glasses of water a day.

The days of sitting down and eating all your meals at home are a thing of the past. Therefore, destressing the eating process means learning to adapt your eating behaviors to our "on-the-run" society. Make a commitment to adhere to your eating plan everywhere. You can do this only if you make sure your foods are portable and convenient and if you are flexible about the types of foods you eat so long as they are High-Quality/Low-Stress Woman Foods.

Here are some ideas on how to prepare for Plan B.

1. At home:

■ Have an emergency breakfast/lunch ready: Keep cans of Ultra Slim-Fast in the refrigerator, packages of Instant Breakfast, and cans of soy protein powder on hand to make smoothies.

■ Cook extra meat when you make dinner. Use this diced for sandwich filling, shredded in a pita, or sliced in a vegetable or pasta salad.

- Use the precleaned and cut-up vegetables and fruits that are available in supermarkets. They do cost more, but they save time and are ready to eat when you are.

- Take twenty minutes to cut up an assortment of vegetables and store them in sealable plastic bowls. You can use these as sandwich stuffings, add them to foods such as omelets, and make salads from them.

- Cut up a colorful assortment of fruit. Fill a smaller container with fruit to draw from throughout the day for snacks and meals.

- Make the best use of frozen entrees available in the freezer section of the supermarket. Clearly, it's always better to eat fresh, whole foods. But under stress and time constraints, frozen foods can suffice. Choose meals that have no more than 3 grams of fat per 100 calories. To boost the nutritional value of your meal, make a few simple additions: a piece of fruit, a glass of juice or milk, a premade salad, or vegetable sticks from the supermarket salad bar.

- Feel free to eat anywhere in your home. Break the rule of eating only at your kitchen or dining room table. If the only way you have time for breakfast at home is to eat it in the bedroom while putting on your clothes, then do it! Don't ever feel guilty about where you nourish yourself!

II. Dashboard dining or in a pinch:

If you're on your way to a meeting and it's lunchtime, you're driving your kids to after-school activities, or you're stuck in traffic, consider these opportunities for creative, flexible eating:

- Eating in your car, or Dashboard Dining, doesn't have to be a disaster. Instead, come fully prepared with your Eating Emergency Kit (EEK). If you spend a great deal of time in your car, it is wise to load up your EEK so that you are always prepared. Fill a cooler with fruit; individual cans of tuna; reduced-fat string cheese; baby carrots; energy bars (e.g., Spirutein, Gensoy, Luna, Essentials); one or two whole wheat pita pockets; an eight-ounce bottle of water; a juice box; sandwich bags filled with a mixture of whole grain cereals (your own trail mix), pretzels, and fat-free granola; a box of raisins; nonfat yogurt; and dried fruit. Don't forget to pack plastic spoons, straws, and napkins.

- For those with less predictable daily schedules, your EEK will be an adult version of a child's lunch box. Purchase a temperature-regulated lunch container so you can bring your own food and avoid missing meals or snacks.
- If you're going to miss dinner because you'll be on your way to an activity, make another sandwich when you pack your lunch and eat on the run.
- If a quick bite of something fattening is the only option, use your head. A slice of pizza becomes almost healthy if you remove all the melted cheese topping. If a drive-in fast-food place is where the family wants to stop, don't panic. Order a salad, a plain baked potato, or a grilled chicken sandwich (hold the sauce).

III. When you travel:

- On pleasure trips, add activity to your life. Bring your tennis racket, carry a jump rope, bring your workout clothes, sneakers, and swimsuit, and definitely check out the fitness center. At certain resorts, you can rent sports equipment such as golf clubs. Take a brisk walk and explore your surroundings.
- Bring food with you, like dried fruit, nonfat dry milk for coffee (in a small sandwich bag), sandwich bags filled with dry cereal or pretzels, granola bars, and energy bars.
- On business trips, try to order a room service breakfast (cereal and extra fruit, or egg-white or **Egg B**eater omelet with toast and extra fruit). Take the extra fruit, which is usually a banana or apple, with you in your briefcase just in case your midmorning snack is delayed. That way you'll have an alternative to the meeting room pastries.
- Whether on a business or pleasure trip, never forget to have your midmorning or midafternoon snack, even if you are attending a meeting or event. Simply reach into your

purse or briefcase for an energy bar and quietly munch on
it. If you skip the snack, you may be overly hungry for the
next meal, which increases your psychological, as well as
physiological, stress. A key to destressing is to honor your
snacks as much as your main meals.

IV. At restaurants:

- **Be prepared for large portions. Order soup and salad first.
  You might not even want an entree. Eat only half of the
  pasta or rice on your plate. Or if this is dinner, eliminate
  all starch (pasta, rice, potato, bread).**
- **Know the type of restaurant and what sort of foods will be
  available. If it's Italian, choose pasta with marinara sauce
  (red sauce without meat) rather than with a cream sauce.
  Be assertive and ask for baked, broiled, or grilled meats,
  chicken, or fish.**
- **If you are eating at a Tex-Mex restaurant, bypass the tor-
  tilla chips and cheese and stick to the salsa, fresh and
  steamed vegetables, baked, broiled, and grilled meats,
  chicken, and fish. Ask for wraps that are baked, not fried.**
- **At Chinese restaurants, try steamed vegetable dumplings
  or soup as an appetizer. Choose steamed rice rather than
  fried. Steer clear of fried entrees such as sweet-and-sour
  shrimp or chicken.**
- **If you have to eat dinner later than usual, eat a balanced
  snack (for instance, repeat your midafternoon snack)
  when you would normally have had dinner; then you won't
  be as hungry when you get to the restaurant.**
- **Restaurants have also become more amenable to serving
  half portions of food. It doesn't hurt to ask.**
- **Ask the waiter to put half the entree in a take-out container and then have it for lunch the next day.**
- **As for desserts, order one if you really want it and have a
  bite or two, then offer it to your dining companions.**

Deb found that once she was out of the dieting mind-set, desserts
weren't so important to her. "I would go out and order the highest
calorie thing as if they were leaving the planet tomorrow—even if

they weren't necessarily what I really wanted. Now I'll pick a vegetable dish or a plain fruit thing for dessert. I can't get over what I've been missing."

Plan B is real life. It's the best intentions colliding with the unexpected. So many women have sat across from me in my office and said, "But, Dr. Peeke, I forgot to bring my snacks to the office." "I'm not a breakfast person." "I didn't have time for lunch." "I'm a failure . . . I can't do this . . . I cheated. . . ."

What should you do if you don't follow your plan one day? *Regroup*. Don't beat yourself up, tell yourself you're a failure and all those other old negative diet speak clichés, which lead to nothing more than Toxic Stress. Instead, understand that life is full of opportunities to regroup.

Plan A is great when our days go according to plan and we don't encounter the dips, twists, and turns that life inevitably throws our way. A sick child in the morning, a meeting that goes through lunch, traffic jams, after-school activities that run through dinnertime are just some of the things that can make the best-laid plans a fantasy.

What do we do? Throw all our efforts away? Give up and decide that there's no use? Give in to stress and let it intoxicate our bodies and minds?

Women are extremists. We are perfectionists and expect ourselves to live up to standards we would never impose on our husbands or children. This type of thinking results in our losing control over our eating, our health, and our lives. As we showed earlier, women under stress reach for snacks that are loaded with fat, sugar, and calories. This makes us feel guilty, angry, put-upon, and hassled. Let's stop being so hard on ourselves, stop thinking we have to be perfect, and become more flexible.

We must learn to be more resilient—to bend, within limits; to accept life's challenges and adapt to them without self-destructive eating.

So we turn to Plan B. Plan A and Plan B are interchangeable. You don't have to follow one or the other. Plan B is what you use when life throws you a curveball. Plan B is your secret weapon to keep yourself Stress-Resilient. The key to successfully implementing Plan B is to be prepared, be flexible, and be creative.

"But Dr. Peeke, *what if* . . .

. . . I woke up late and have to be at work for a meeting."

Fine. *Then you* . . .

. . . Slide into Plan B: Grab a can of Ultra SlimFast from the refrigerator to Dashboard Dine in your car on your way to work. Use your Eating Emergency Kit and have some yogurt and fruit on your way to work.

"Well, that sounds easy. But *what if* . . .

. . . My child is sick in the morning, my kids miss the bus, or the baby-sitter doesn't show?"

Not a problem. *Then you* . . .

. . . Have your breakfast at home, pack a lunch since you won't have time to go out because you're so late to work, and Dashboard Dine on baby carrots or fruit on the way to work in the midmorning.

"*What if* . . .

. . . I'll be getting home late from work and have to take the kids to soccer practice?"

Don't panic. *Then you* . . .

. . . Pack a sandwich and put it in the cooler for dinner at the practice. Round out your dinner with other goodies in your cooler: nonfat yogurt, baby carrots, fruit.

"*What if* . . .

. . . I'm starved. The midafternoon munchies have hit and I succumb to a handful of cookies?"

Okay. It happens. *Then you* . . .

. . . Still eat dinner, but make it smaller and take a walk before or after you eat.

"*What if* . . .

. . . It's after dinner and my appetite kicks in?"

Check to see if you're under stress. Remember, it is now the CortiZone time and you are more vulnerable to stress eating. Remind yourself that what you have is probably not true hunger; instead you probably have appetite, or "I want." *Then you* . . .

. . . Have a snack including protein, such as one or two pieces of string cheese, yogurt, a fruit smoothie, or even a cup of cereal with milk.

"*What if* . . .

. . . I have a dinner engagement at 8 P.M., it's 6 P.M., and I haven't eaten since three, my midafternoon snack time?"

Then you . . .

. . . Have a snack with protein, fat, and carbohydrate, since it is three hours after your midafternoon snack. Remember that the later you eat, the lighter you should eat. Therefore, you will be eating smaller portions at dinner, primarily salad, vegetables, and protein. This means passing on the appetizer, moving the bread basket away from your plate, tasting and savoring your food, not gulping and overconsuming, and taking the leftovers home in a doggie bag so you can have them for lunch the next day.

"*What if . . .*

. . . I'm out for dinner and I really want dessert?"

Then you . . .

. . . Order it! But be sure to share it with as many people as you can. Taste and savor and thoroughly enjoy it. Remember, the price you will have to pay for that dessert is increased physical activity to burn it off. If you haven't already had your exercise that day, you have to do so the next day.

"*What if . . .*

. . . I was in a meeting that lasted all afternoon, and I missed my midafternoon snack. Now I'm on my way home and I'm famished."

Do not do a fast-food "drive-buy." *Instead, you . . .*

. . . Open your Eating Emergency Kit and have a snack of pretzels and reduced-fat string cheese or nonfat yogurt with a sandwich bag of cereal and a piece of fruit or an energy bar.

The key to successful Plan B eating is learning that many times you will not be able to eat exactly as you planned. Furthermore, your eating circumstances (in your car, running to a meeting, sitting on a bus, waiting in an airport) may not be optimal and as enjoyable as if you were living your Plan A routine. Accept the fact that Plan B is a compromise. Avoid the perfectionist's tendency to cling to Plan A and to fear leaving the safe harbor of a regular routine. You will learn that as you become more masterful at making the transition from A to B and back, you will also become better at regrouping in other parts of your life.

■ It's All About Portions

Keep in mind that it is almost impossible, outside of a food science laboratory, to keep track of your calories perfectly. Therefore, I am much more concerned with your portions. For women over forty, watching portions is imperative. This is because even the fittest over-forty woman must get used to eating less due to declining metabolism. Therefore, it becomes more critical to be visually aware of how much you eat. Read the USDA labels on the food you buy, consider portions based on the content of the meal.

I always say that if women read the USDA levels as closely and thoroughly as they read clothing labels in a department store, half the problem of overeating would be solved. Study food labels as you would a garment label, and you'll be in better control of your food portions.

Keep in mind that "servings" and "portions" are not the same things. A serving of a food is an amount determined by the USDA to calculate its nutritional value in accordance with the USDA food pyramid. A portion is the amount of a food you eat at a single sitting. A portion may be one or multiple servings. For example, a USDA serving of a bagel equals one-half bagel. If you eat an entire bagel, you will have consumed two servings. As the USDA recommends six to eleven servings per day from the bread, cereal, rice, and pasta group, you have now consumed two of these servings.

In the morning, as an experiment, measure out your cereal serving as dictated by the food label on the carton. You may be amazed that it is less than what you had expected. Pour the measuring cup's serving size into your cereal bowl and memorize what it looks like. You see, you didn't need to become a calorie mathematician; all you needed to do was to remember visually what a serving size looks like. You only need to practice with your measuring cup a few times before you get the jist of it.

Next, take your measuring cup and fill to one-half cup with cooked pasta or rice. Place that in the middle of a plate. Now fill the measuring cup to one cup with cooked pasta or rice and place that in the middle of another plate. Stare at these and memorize what they look like. You should know that most typical restaurant portions include three to five cups of rice or pasta.

Since most restaurant portions are man-sized servings, a woman is left on her own to create High-Quality/Low-Stress Woman Food portions. You will know what that portion is by first practicing at home and learning exactly how much half of a cup of pasta or rice really looks like. If you think it doesn't look like much on your plate, add two to four cups of steamed or grilled vegetables. Now you have a large plate of healthy vegetables with an appropriate Woman Food portion of pasta or rice.

When you are having cereal or soup, use a smaller-size bowl than you typically use. Further, when you go to a buffet, select a small plate and it will be more difficult to overeat.

Now, let's consider a treat item like ice cream. Look on the USDA label of the ice cream carton and read what a single serving amounts to in quantity. Scoop one-half cup of ice cream into a measuring cup and then place it in a bowl. If you use a large bowl, the serving will look tiny. For your delectable treats in Woman Food portions of one-half-cup to one-cup serving sizes, I suggest using a small bowl or a sorbet glass. Add fruit, such as berries, on top, and you have a beautiful dessert to enjoy in a Woman Food portion.

An average serving of poultry or lean meat for a woman is anywhere from three to four ounces. Restaurants often serve twice that. Again, it might be helpful, just once, to weigh your foods just as a learning experience to understand what three and four ounces look like. Realize also that, with fish, you can eat up to twice the number of ounces as you would with lean meat or poultry, and therefore your portion can be so much bigger—fish is a real winner in terms of protein.

A problem occurs when women deal with foods that do not come in single-size servings. Women, therefore, must create their own Woman Food-size servings. For instance, bread comes in a loaf. Read the label and realize that a woman-size portion for a sandwich is two pieces; for breakfast, one or two pieces. Once you enter the CortiZone, stress tends to stimulate a limitless consumption of that loaf of bread. Be aware that during the CortiZone, you must be prepared to eat Woman Food portion sizes. During the CortiZone, increasing stress and decreasing focus make you more vulnerable to disregard portion and serving size as you desperately seek anesthesia from food. Therefore, a key to success in navigating the CortiZone is to be prepared, both mentally and specifically at mealtimes, to know what Woman Food portions are and to live with them. Entering the CortiZone without paying attention to portion size is a guarantee of weight gain at any age.

Table 7-2 shows Plan A guidelines for daily food servings. I have used the classic USDA Food Guide Pyramid and made adjustments to increase the servings of fruits and vegetables. Also, I have specifically noted servings for meats, fish, and legumes.

Table 7-2. **Plan A Guidelines for Daily Food Servings**

In conjunction with daily physical activity

Type of Food	Serving Size	Number of Servings
Whole grains (bread, cereal, rice, pasta)	1 slice bread, ½ bagel, ½ cup cooked pasta, rice, or cereal, 1 tortilla	6 or more per day
Vegetables	1 piece, ½ cup cooked or canned, 1 cup raw, 6 ounces juice	6–8 per day
Fruits	1 piece, ½ cup cooked or canned, 1 cup raw, 6 ounces juice	5–6 per day
Milk, yogurt, and cheese (low-fat)	1 cup milk, 1 ounce cheese, 1 cup yogurt	2–3 per day
Meat, poultry, fish, dry beans, eggs, and nuts or seeds	¾ cup cooked beans, 3 ounces fish, 3 ounces skinless poultry breast, 1 egg, 3 ounces red meat, ⅓ ounce nuts or seeds, 10–15 nuts	2 per day Fish: 3–4 per week, Red meat: 3 per month, Poultry: 3–5 per week, Dry beans: 1–2 per day, Nuts or seeds: 1–2 per day, Eggs: 4 per week
Fats and oils: Olive or canola oil Other vegetable oils	1 tablespoon	Up to 2 per day Up to 1 per day
Refined, processed sugars		Minimize or avoid

■ Stress Profile Eating

Now it's time to put into practice Plan A eating routines for each stress profile. First, I offer examples of eating in a Stress-Resilient way over the course of a week. Generally speaking, each day's food composition adheres to the classic recommendations for carbohydrates, protein, and fat, as previously described. The caloric content of each diet is approximately 1,500 calories per day. Clearly, make the appropriate adjustments based on your own weight and activity level, as described earlier.

Stress-Resilient	
Day 1:	
Breakfast	Egg white omelet, whole wheat toast, fresh orange, glass of skim milk
Midmorning snack	Fresh fruit with low-fat cottage cheese
Lunch	Whole wheat pita stuffed with drained water-packed tuna, chopped tomatoes, and black olives, baby carrots, fresh plums
Midafternoon snack	Sliced apple with reduced-fat peanut butter on wheat bread
Dinner	Grilled salmon, green beans sprinkled with lemon pepper, tossed salad with Italian dressing, nonfat yogurt with fruit
Day 2:	
Breakfast	Whole wheat toast topped with low-fat cottage cheese and cinnamon and broiled until bubbly, sliced peaches
Midmorning snack	Cereal-fruit bar with nonfat yogurt
Lunch	Pasta salad with vegetables and cooked fish or poultry seasoned with reduced-fat Italian dressing, whole grain roll, orange wedges (or other fresh fruit)

Midafternoon snack	Reduced-fat cheese sticks and pretzels or saltines
Dinner	Shrimp kabobs, spinach-and-mushroom salad, fresh pineapple (Marinate shrimp in a mixture of olive oil, dill, and lemon juice, and put on a skewer with cherry or grape tomatoes, onion slices, and green and red peppers. Grill over hot coals.)

Day 3:

Breakfast	Nonfat yogurt, toasted English muffin with fruit spread, cantaloupe
Midmorning snack	Baby carrots with reduced-calorie dressing, reduced-fat string cheese
Lunch	Pea soup, brown rice salad (cooked and chilled brown rice, cut-up vegetables, and dressing of choice), wheat crackers, sliced peaches and strawberries (or other fresh fruit), skim milk
Midafternoon snack	Peanut butter on wheat crackers, banana
Dinner	Barbecued chicken, cooked whole baby carrots seasoned with a sprinkle of dill, boiled whole new potatoes, (yes, it's all right to have a dense starch at night as a treat once in a while), fresh melon cubes (or other fresh fruit)

Day 4:

Breakfast	Whole grain cereal with fruit, skim milk
Midmorning snack	Nonfat yogurt, dried apple rings and apricot halves
Lunch	Vegetable soup, cottage cheese and cucumber sandwich on pumpernickel bread, sliced fresh pears
Midafternoon snack	Reduced-fat string cheese with pretzels, wheat crackers, or reduced-fat microwave popcorn
Dinner	Raw vegetable salad with chicken, fresh fruit, skim milk

Day 5:

Breakfast	Smoothie (made with nonfat yogurt, skim milk, and fruit), whole grain toast with fruit spread
Midmorning snack	Low-fat bran muffin, skim milk
Lunch	Chopped chicken on pumpernickel bread with fresh spinach leaves, tomato, and Dijon mustard
Midafternoon snack	Cut-up vegetables and reduced-fat cheese with low-calorie dip, crackers
Dinner	Sole cooked in orange or grapefruit juice, steamed broccoli spears seasoned with lemon juice, broiled tomato halves

Day 6:

Breakfast	Scrambled egg whites, whole wheat toast with all-fruit spread, fresh orange wedges, skim milk
Midmorning snack	Fruit with low-fat cottage cheese
Lunch	Black bean soup, broiled tomato and reduced-fat cheese sandwich on oatmeal bread, fresh pink grapefruit sections
Midafternoon snack	Apple slices with peanut butter
Dinner	Sautéed tofu and vegetables seasoned with soy sauce and ginger, brown rice, fresh melon wedges

Day 7:

Breakfast	Oatmeal with raisins and skim milk, orange juice
Midmorning snack	Granola bar, nonfat yogurt
Lunch	Tabouli (Lebanese wheat salad), nonfat yogurt, kiwifruit and strawberries
Midafternoon snack	Tomato or vegetable juice, reduced-fat string cheese, wheat crackers
Dinner	Broiled scrod, steamed spinach with lemon wedges, baked sweet potato

■ Beginning the Journey as a Stress Overeater or Stress Undereater

It is important to recognize that the Stress Overeater and Stress Undereater will approach this journey toward more healthy eating differently. The Stress Undereater tends to be rigidly in control of her eating and is generally terrorized by the eating process. Stress Undereaters respond well to smaller, more frequent meals. The Stress Undereater's eating plan, therefore, includes suggestions for a less stressful, more healthy eating routine. Rather than her old Plan A of caloric restriction, her new Plan A includes a constant exposure, throughout the day, to healthy food in quantities she can learn to appreciate. On the other hand, the Stress Overeater must strive to become an expert at portion control as well as planned eating on a regular basis throughout the day. Stress Overeaters are also terrified of, as well as frustrated by, eating in general. Introducing Stress Overeaters to food as a safe and healthy fuel will destress their eating process.

Both Stress Overeaters and Stress Undereaters need to keep their Plan A simple and well planned as they enter the CortiZone. During the CortiZone, the Stress Undereater tends to stop or severely restrict her eating. On the other hand, from 3 P.M. on, Stress Overeaters are vulnerable to using food as an anesthetic for coping with their increasing fatigue, decreasing focus, and frustration with the day's stresses. Once Stress Overeaters and Stress Undereaters become comfortable with their new Plan A, they can begin to practice designing Plan B to implement when stresses in their lives interrupt their Plan A routines. Arming themselves with an Eating Emergency Kit as well as putting deliberate thought and preparation into eating during the CortiZone will allow all the stress profiles to make the transition into the CortiZone, relying on a well-thought-out Plan B when necessary.

Sample stress-neutralizing menus for Stress Overeaters and Stress Undereaters follow on pages 176 and 177.

Regardless of your stress profile, if you are over forty, healthy eating in the twenty-first century means taking vitamin and mineral supplements along with your whole foods. Science has helped us understand what a perimenopausal body and mind need to stay well.

Stress Overeater

Day 1:

Breakfast	½ cup cereal, fresh fruit, skim milk
Midmorning snack	Reduced-fat string cheese, 6 saltines
Lunch	Sandwich, carrot and celery sticks, fresh fruit, skim milk
Midafternoon snack	Yogurt, fresh fruit, graham crackers
Dinner	3 ounces poultry or fish, at least 2 servings of vegetables (1 cooked, 1 raw), fresh fruit

Day 2:

Breakfast	1 egg (hard-cooked, poached, or scrambled), 1 slice whole wheat toast with 1 tablespoon reduced-sugar jam, baked apple, skim milk
Midmorning snack	Nonfat yogurt, fresh fruit
Lunch	Corn tortilla filled with black beans, corn, tomatoes, and shredded lettuce and seasoned with vinaigrette, cucumber slices, vegetable juice
Midafternoon snack	Low-fat cottage cheese, fresh fruit, 6 saltines
Dinner	3 ounces sole, zucchini and tomatoes, shredded cabbage, carrots and onion tossed with reduced-calorie French dressing

Day 3:

Breakfast	Nonfat yogurt mixed with low-fat granola, citrus fruit cup
Midmorning snack	Cereal-fruit bar, skim milk
Lunch	Tuna canned in water (3-ounce can), wheat roll, carrot or celery sticks or pepper rings
Midafternoon snack	6 saltines, ¼ cup bean dip (made from fat-free refried beans seasoned with onion, garlic, and chili powders)
Dinner	Vegetable soup (no cream soups), relish plate, roll, fresh fruit

Stress Undereater

Day 1:

Breakfast	Ultra Slim-Fast shake in a thermos to sip throughout morning
Midmorning snack	Sandwich bag with trail mix to munch throughout morning: low-fat granola, dried fruit, nuts
Lunch	Sandwich with chicken, turkey, or ham, carrot and celery sticks, piece of fruit
Midafternoon snack	Spirutein bar
Dinner	Frozen entree, tossed salad with dressing, fresh fruit, skim milk

Day 2:

Breakfast	½ peanut butter/apple slice sandwich (prepare the evening before, cut in quarters for easy eating throughout the morning), fruit juice
Midmorning snack	½ peanut butter/apple slice sandwich
Lunch	Yogurt, graham crackers, fresh fruit
Midafternoon snack	Reduced-fat string cheese, crackers, baby carrots, tomato or vegetable juice
Dinner	Vegetable soup, ½ whole wheat pita filled with ricotta cheese (made from skim milk), packaged shredded vegetables seasoned with reduced-calorie vinaigrette, fresh fruit, skim milk

Day 3:

Breakfast	Cereal-fruit bar, nonfat yogurt, fresh fruit
Midmorning snack	Fresh fruit
Lunch	Low-fat cottage cheese, relish plate (with vegetables and hard-cooked egg), fresh fruit, saltines
Midafternoon snack	Nutrition bar
Dinner	Broiled fish, snow peas or other green vegetable, steamed baby carrots, fresh fruit or dried fruit compote

■ Speaking of Supplements

In a perfect world, we would be able to obtain all the essential nutrients from our daily diets. However, nutritionists have found that the majority of Americans' diets fall considerably short of the basic requirements for sustaining good health. Meal skipping, nutrient-empty fast foods and snack items, and chronic dieting all result in a depletion of the body's stores of vitamins and minerals.

In addition, the human body is constantly under biological stress. It is physiologically stressful for the body to absorb environmental pollution (e.g., ultraviolet radiation, someone else's cigarette smoke, car exhaust). Life is a constant threat to the immune system, which needs to fend off and repair damage done everyday.

Biological stress also occurs when we eat highly processed and chemically enhanced foods. It is estimated that the American adult is exposed to approximately 10,000 new chemicals each year in processed foods. Dyes, preservatives, and chemically modified foods (e.g., transfatty acids in margarine and oils) cause cellular stress in the body. In addition, fake fats (e.g., Olestra) as well as the newer diet supplements (e.g., Orlistat) often cause gastrointestinal stress. (I tell my patients if they really want potato chips to go ahead and eat a few real chips, rather than eat an entire bag of "fat-free" chips.)

The damage to the immune system is manifested as increased oxidation at the cellular level.

What exactly does that mean? Oxidation is the process by which cells are challenged by any stress and, as a consequence, break down. One result of the oxidative process is the generation of free radicals, which can then circulate and wreak havoc within the body. These radicals are produced when a cell is stressed. The key is to neutralize the radicals with antioxidants.

Vitamins and minerals help your cells by providing antioxidants, which neutralize the oxidation process and help protect the integrity of the cells. Antioxidants are found in many foods, primarily fruits and vegetables. Consider fruits and vegetables to be huge bank accounts from which you can always withdraw an endless amount of antioxidant currency to stay healthy!

As we age, our cells need more help to stay fit. They've been working hard for at least forty years, and their ability to fend off oxidation is becoming more and more difficult. Therefore, after the age of forty, it is wise to supplement your healthy diet with antioxidants to optimize health. Table 7-3 lists the basic daily vitamin and mineral supplements.

Here are some tips:

- **Buy a simple multivitamin and mineral supplement from your grocery or pharmacy. The major brands (e.g., Centrum, Bayer, Theragram) will usually do the trick. Avoid spending lots of money on designer vitamins, which are usually overloaded with high doses of these ingredients. There is no proof that taking megadoses of these vitamins and minerals is of significant benefit to your health.**
- **Vitamin E is the most prominent of the fat-soluble vitamins. It is a powerful antioxidant, and studies have shown its benefits in preventing cardiovascular disease. Remember that heart disease is still the number one killer of women in midlife. More than 200,000 women die each year from heart disease. You need to protect your heart as**

Table 7-3. Recommended Over-Forty Dietary Supplements

Multivitamin and mineral* supplement

Vitamin E: 400 IU (up to 800 IU if heart disease is present or risk is high)

Selenium: 100 mcg (up to 200 mcg if immune system is compromised)

Vitamin C: 250 mg (up to 500 mg if at high risk for heart disease, or 1,000 mg if heart disease is present)

Vitamin B: complex

Calcium: 1,000–1,500 mg

Vitamin D: 200 IU (only if not included in multivitamin or calcium supplement)

Omega (fish) oil: 1,000 mg

Flaxseed oil: 1,000 mg

---

*Multivitamin should contain 100 percent of established value of vitamins and minerals.

well as your immune system! After age forty, women need to take 400 IU of vitamin E and then increase this to 800 IU after the age of fifty. If, in your forties, you are at very high risk of heart disease or already have it, increasing to 800 IU is appropriate. Remember that vitamin E is also a mild blood thinner, and always check with your doctor before beginning any supplement to make certain that you are not at risk of certain complications.

■ Selenium is a powerful boost to the immune system. It makes the immune function stronger. Studies have shown that it appears to prevent cancer, especially colon cancer. It is also good for anyone with a medical condition involving immune system compromise, such as any autoimmune disorder (e.g., rheumatoid arthritis) or even cancer. If you have any of these conditions, it is helpful to increase your dose to 200 micrograms daily.

■ Vitamin B complex contains all of the essential B vitamins, including folate, which is helpful in preventing the rise of homocysteine, an amino acid implicated in heart disease. Make certain your doctor runs a blood test for your homocysteine level next time you go in for a checkup, as you may need additional folate if it is elevated.

■ Calcium should be a daily supplement for all women over the age of forty. Don't wait for menopause to take place in your fifties. Make certain to get a bone density scan no later than age forty-five so that you know where you stand. It is important to buy a supplement that has a high level of bioavailability (is absorbed well by the body). Calcium carbonate is absorbed least easily; calcium citrate is much better. Try to get a supplement fortified with vitamin D, as many of them now are. The highest bioavailability actually comes from a compound called calcium hydroxyappetite, which is now available in pharmacies.

■ Vitamin D doesn't need to be taken as a supplement unless you are not getting enough in your diet or you are not being exposed to the sun for at least fifteen minutes every day. Vitamin D aids in the absorption of calcium. Most calcium and multivitamin supplements contain the required amount.

■ The omega-3 fatty acids found in fish oil have been shown to prevent as well as treat heart disease. Having at least three servings of fish per week helps get these important oils into your system. After the age of forty, I recommend augmenting your dietary intake with 1,000 milligrams of fish oil. If you have heart disease or are at high risk of it, you can increase this to 3,000 milligrams per day under your doctor's supervision.

■ Flaxseed oil contains the fatty acids that are essential to maintaining immune function. As you age, it is more important to include this immune-boosting supplement in your diet.

■ Destressing the Perimenopause with Food

Because my medical practice and research have been devoted to women's health issues, I have found that there are many foods that are uniquely beneficial to a woman's health during menopause.

Just as chicken soup made us feel better when we had the flu as children, many foods can soothe your symptoms as your hormones begin to fluctuate. Depression, hot flashes, night sweats, and other discomforts can often be lessened with dietary intervention. Table 7-4 lists some helpful suggestions.

By now you have had an opportunity to combine your regrouping skills with healthy eating. Next, you will learn why physical activity is the currency with which you pay for the food you eat each day.

Table 7-4. **Perimenopausal Symptomatology and Solutions**

Symptom	Solution	Sources
Fatigue	Eat iron-rich foods.	Meats and poultry
Irritability, memory loss, depression	Take a vitamin B complex: B vitamins are essential to normal functioning of the nervous system.	
Indigestion	Have small, frequent meals; eat low-fat foods and avoid fried foods and lunch meats.	
Hot flashes	Eat soy products.	Soy milk, soybeans, tofu
	Consume foods containing vitamin E. Some studies show that vitamin E supplementation, up to 400 IU twice daily, is helpful.	Wheat germ, safflower oil, whole grain breads and cereals, walnuts, filberts, almonds, sunflower seeds
Sweating	Eat soy products.	Soy milk, soybeans, tofu
Water retention	Consume the majority of your calories and carbohydrates early in the day before dinner.	
Headaches	Some studies support increasing dietary magnesium.	Nuts (almonds, cashews, walnuts), tofu, leafy dark green vegetables (e.g., spinach), wheat germ

Constipation	Eat high-fiber foods; include 20 to 35 grams of fiber in your diet every day. Drink plenty of water. Exercise.	Bran cereals and breads, whole grain cereals and breads, fruits and vegetables, legumes (beans, peas, lentils)
Carbohydrate cravings	Have small, frequent meals. When you eat carbohydrates, choose higher-fiber foods.	Whole wheat bread, whole grain cereals, oatmeal
Reduced metabolic rate	Do strength training.	
Dry skin, hair, mouth	Drink 8 glasses of water each day.	
Increased risk of heart disease	Eat soy products.	Soy milk, soybeans, tofu
	Include omega-3 fatty acids in your diet.	Salmon, mackerel, tuna
	Decrease your intake of saturated fat.	(No-nos: heavily marbled meats, cream, whole milk and whole milk products)
	Eat foods high in antioxidants (vitamin C).	Broccoli, cauliflower, green pepper, cantaloupe, oranges, grapefruit, kiwifruit, strawberries
	Eat foods high in antioxidants (vitamin E).	Wheat germ, safflower oil, whole grain breads and cereals, peanuts, walnuts, filberts, almonds, sunflower seeds

	Eat foods high in antioxidants (beta-carotene).	Carrots, broccoli, sweet potatoes, spinach, cantaloupe
	Exercise.	
	Stop smoking.	
Sleep disturbances	Don't eat after dinner, especially not right before going to bed.	
Urinary tract infections	Drink 8 glasses of water per day. Drink cranberry juice.	
Decreased bone mass	Exercise. Consume more calcium; use supplements if necessary. Take vitamin D supplements.	Milk and dairy products

Template Three
Stress-Resilient Physical Activity

8 The Double Whammy: Stress and Inactivity During Menopause

Some women over forty dread the thought of exercise. Others are confused. "Why," they ask, "is it so important for a woman to take the time to exercise every day?" Does her life depend upon it? Yes.

The majority of us are not athletes, nor are we models, actresses, or dancers. More options are available today for women: We are teachers, administrators, secretaries, computer programmers, businesswomen, nurses, doctors, and lawyers as well as daughters, sisters, wives, and mothers. We currently own 38 percent of all U.S. businesses. Women now outpace men in college degrees earned (56 percent to 44 percent in 1999) and we are expected to take a similar lead in graduate degrees earned.

But our professional or academic success stories are often clouded by personal disappointments about our bodies brought on by stress eating and lack of self-care. One of my patients once said to me, "I am a very successful executive. I made all the right schooling and career decisions. My income and my self-worth come from what

- Determine Your Fitness Level

- Some Is Better Than None: Accrue Exercise and Burn Toxic Weight Throughout the Day

- Stress Hormone Management Through Aerobic Activity

my mind can produce at work and home. However, my body is usually pushed to the background."

While we focused on our professional, academic, community, and family obligations and achievements, we forgot the needs of our bodies. We need to strike a balance in our lives. We need to finally accept that our bodies are an *essential part* of the equation of our success in life.

As women in our forties and fifties, we are unique because we were never taught that exercise should be an integral part of our lives. We were rarely even instructed on how to stay active and exercise once we left school. Today, we are realizing that our bodies have distinct needs. Our muscles need to be strengthened. Our tendons and ligaments need to be flexible. Why? To stay healthy and active for many years to come.

The National Institute of Aging has now determined that what we used to think of as symptoms *of aging* (easy fatigue, memory impairment, loss of strength and flexibility, declining muscle mass, aching joints) are actually symptoms *of disuse*!

Men and women had been led to believe that fifty signaled a natural decline in physical as well as mental function. We were wrong! A twenty-first-century American woman can be expected to live to at least eighty, an increase of thirty-three years since 1990! American men will live to seventy-seven years and beyond. Now, fifty represents a great time to regroup and get ready for thirty more years of a full and active life. For that matter, it is predicted that by the year 2050 there will be more than one million centenarians (one-hundred-year-olds) alive. If you're currently fifty, this could be you.

Today's women need to scrap the old "you don't need exercise" messages they heard as they grew up. Girls in our generation, in fact, were often discouraged from participating in vigorous physical activity. Remember how easily you could be excused from gym class because it was "that time of the month"? Sex role stereotypes formed early in life often dictate future activity levels. Sadly, this means that many forty- to fifty-five-year-old women may never achieve their physical fitness potential.

We also grew up in a culture that saw strength as masculine and a small, soft, frail body as feminine. The Audrey Hepburn silhouette comes to mind. Some of us were lucky and had great experiences with physical activity in school. Our athletic accomplishments often led to a great sense of self-esteem and were carried with us as metaphors for achievements as we became adults. However, there might have been negative experiences growing up. I know all about the embarrassment of exposing one's body to the world. I remember ridiculous get-ups we had to prance around in for PE class—the blue jumpers that not even the cheerleaders looked good in.

We had calisthenics in the 1950s. There were Jack LaLanne and Bonnie Pruden, wearing tights and doing sit-ups. And, of course, those Air Force exercises. When Jane Fonda opened her first aerobics studio in Los Angeles in the 1970s, millions of women began doing the "grapevine" to the thumping beat of disco. Then came a flotilla of fitness experts, from Richard Simmons to Cindy Crawford. Feeling the burn.

Despite all that, today's billion-dollar exercise industry is relatively young. For example, Weight Watchers didn't add physical activity to its plan until the 1990s. Although there is a vast increase in sports participation by female students, up from 300,000 in 1971 to around 2.5 million today, many women who came of age in the 1960s never participated in organized activities like swimming, softball, basketball, soccer, or field hockey teams. Now all of a sudden, after never having been taught how to exercise or lift weights, perimenopausal women are faced with the dilemma of how to whip themselves into shape—seemingly, instantly.

Banish those thoughts. You are older and wiser and, believe it or not, you can still get healthy, active, and fit at any age! Keep in mind that exercising after forty is no longer about competition or looking cute in a leotard. This isn't about the buns of steel or a six-pack abdomen. This is about using exercise as a way to destress your daily mental wear and tear, decrease your perimenopausal symptoms, get fit and firm, and guarantee high-quality living into the twenty-first century.

As I have mentioned in Part One, women often live in a state of mind-body dissociation. Actually, the body is a whole being, a totality.

Candace Pert, Ph.D., the internationally acclaimed molecular biologist and author of *Molecules of Emotion*, once noted that the body is actually "dense mind," and that mind and body are inextricably linked. Neglecting one hurts the other.

Movement can be fun. Exercise can make you feel strong. Sweat can give you a true feeling of accomplishment. Working out is something you will want to commit to doing every day *to take care of your body*.

■ Exercise and Our Perimenopausal Experience

We know that perimenopause is a shock to your system. In fact, it takes a woman's body an entire year to adjust to the shifting hormones. This natural transition is made more difficult by our unnatural sedentary lifestyles. As we have learned, our metabolisms slow down with age. By the time we turn forty, we are facing our third major decrease. In addition, our metabolisms might have been subjected to additional decreases due to years of chronic dieting that stripped us of muscle mass. Our inactivity leaves us no options to counter these effects.

We are confronting the effects of the shifting hormones of perimenopause: fat is now gravitating toward the abdomen, producing our menopot, piling on excessive fat inside our abdomen and leaving us more vulnerable to Toxic Weight. We may suffer from other common symptoms associated with menopause: hot flashes, anxiety, depression, declining energy, fatigue, and/or difficulty sleeping, declining self-esteem, problems with memory or concentration. Believe it or not, exercise is the solution to all of this!

■ The Triple Threat

But what happens when we add Toxic Stress to the combination of perimenopause and inactivity? It's a triple threat to the system.

Perimenopausal women who have no physical activity in their lives are extremely vulnerable to the Toxic Weight that results from Toxic Stress. They have no physical outlet for their daily stresses. Instead, the stresses accumulate, elevating levels of circulating cortisol, and stimulating abdominal fat cells to continually store more fat, which puts women on the path to the metabolic syndrome.

Deb's Story

Take Deb for example. You may remember her story from the Nutrition Template. At forty-three and on the cusp of perimenopause, Deb suffered from horrible fatigue as well as low energy and self-esteem. She was a lifelong Stress Overeater, and her sedentary lifestyle and stress eating had led her to an unhealthy weight and bulging waistline. She frequently suffered from minor illnesses and, having been recently diagnosed with high blood pressure, began to worry about her family history of disease.

Deb accepted exercise as necessary to remove her Toxic Weight. She currently walks three miles per day and has incorporated strength training twice a week into her Plan A. During challenging days, she regroups and will maintain this momentum in a Plan B, where she divides the three miles per day into increments, getting in the walking when she can. Her once-crushing fatigue is a thing of the past. Deb told me, "Life is more fun. I have more energy and stamina to complete my required duties and then have the option of doing fun things without feeling as though it will take a week to recuperate. I love feeling physically empowered." Deb no longer worries about having the energy to run to catch a train.

Her confidence is higher now that she no longer feels it's necessary to "filter everything through the 'fat screen.'" She no longer worries about what other people think of her when dining at a restaurant. Deb is less embarrassed to meet new people and see old friends. She also says she gets sick less often. Her blood pressure is back to normal levels and, perhaps most important, she is no longer terrorized by the possibility of future disease. Deb feels happier and less burdened. Physical activity, "exercise opportunities" she calls it, is something she shares with her husband so they can maintain their well-being and enjoy a long life together.

Finally, Deb began to shed that over-forty weight and get healthier. After having done it for more than a year, Deb

> has found—as so many patients have—that the time she spends exercising has become a sacrosanct time, a time of mental and physical renewal, a point of solace in a busy day. She no longer obsesses about rippling muscles. She knows that exercise is nonnegotiable, a way to optimize the quality of her life.

By now you realize that our original stress response is incomplete in modern life. In other words, we stress but we don't blow it off and that leads to chronic Toxic Stress. Simply put, it is imperative that we *complete* our body's "fight-or-flight" response with the physical activity it expects, thereby breaking the stress-fat cycle. If we don't the only alternative is to stew and chew over stress.

Researchers at the University of Colorado published four studies of animals in 1999 that showed that *moderate exercise can reduce stress,* regardless of its origins. So, you will get and stay in great shape, burning fat and building muscle, while keeping your stress hormones under control.

I now look at gym equipment as "fight-or-flight" simulators and the gym trainers as "fight-or-flight" instructors. It makes it more fun to realize that you are physically letting go and really getting into working off the hassles of the day. This gives your workout the life-saving function of neutralizing your life stresses. It's a way of saying "This really has a role in my life."

Women over forty are at greatest risk for Toxic Stress and, therefore, Toxic Weight. Compounding Toxic Weight, Toxic Stress worsens just as your hormones are beginning to fluctuate in perimenopause, making you even more apt to gain fat in your abdomen. Think of it as a biological seesaw. Your metabolism is decreased and your estrogen is declining while stress hormones are elevated. The result? A bulging waistline—your body has changed from resembling a pear to resembling an apple—and increased risk of disease.

The good news is this cycle is reversible. If stress makes you fat, then becoming more Stress Resilient helps you shed the fat. The key is to get fit. Here's how it works.

You learned in Part One that beta-endorphins neutralize the effects of cortisol. They produce a calming effect, which slows the release of Alarm Hormone and, more important, the appetite-inducing cortisol. Furthermore, they activate the reward system in the brain that leads to feelings of pleasure and fullness. It is easy to see, therefore, how beta-endorphins can also relieve depression, anxiety, and even reduce hot flashes.

I have found that most women experience some levels of depression as they reach the perimenopausal years. There is a solid core of data that shows us that exercise works exquisitely well as an antidepressant. A review of relevant research in 1993 gave support to "the antidepressant, anti-anxiety and mood enhancing effects of exercise programs." In a 1994 review by Dr. Catherine Ross of Ohio State University, she refers to several studies that found both aerobic and weight-lifting exercise lead to a decrease in depression and improved psychological well-being. A 1999 study from Duke University reported that thirty minutes of brisk cardiovascular exercise performed three times per week over the course of sixteen weeks was as effective as antidepressants in relieving symptoms of depression. Study after study shows us that exercise gives us this enhanced sense of well-being.

Physical activity is also a release for anxiety. It bathes the body with soothing brain chemicals, which is nature's way of saying "Relax. The predator is gone." Furthermore, Dr. Fredi Kronenberg of Columbia University reports in a review article that psychological stress is often cited by women as a trigger of hot flashes; and further: that hot flashes can be managed through physical activity.

Many of my patients who were Stress Overeaters have become so enamored of exercise and the way it makes them feel that they literally trade in food for physical activity. Their workouts are their new passions and food has become an afterthought. The Stress Undereaters note that exercise helps to control the relentlessly high levels of stress hormones that plague them with anxiety and nervousness. A brisk walk brings calm and peace.

■ The Basic Effects of Physical Activity

Heart disease is the leading killer of men and women in the United States. The Harvard University School of Public Health has predicted that by the year 2020, it will be the leading cause of death globally. Here's what happens from the moment your heart rate starts to rise to the point—often hours later—where the body is still benefiting from the activity.

Your heart is a muscle that pumps blood throughout your body. That blood carries oxygen, removes waste, and performs other life-sustaining functions. The heart works hard.

When the heart is unfit, it works harder, which can lead to it wearing out. Any part of your body that isn't getting enough blood is going to be tired and painful. So you need to keep that blood pumping. Eating the right kind of food, drinking enough water, and observing other healthy habits will help. But exercise is, as usual, the key.

In this case I mean cardiovascular (which refers to the heart and blood-carrying tubes) exercise. This kind of workout is also called aerobic exercise (not to be confused with "aerobics class," which is just one type of aerobic exercise). Examples of aerobic exercise are walking, biking, rowing, and swimming.

Aerobic exercise gets you breathing hard. It also raises your heart rate, since the heart is getting a healthy workout, too. Aerobic exercise makes your heart fitter. And, yes, it's true, aerobic exercise cuts stress like crazy. Whether you are running after a rambunctious child, sprinting for a bus, or climbing stairs all day, you are helping to break the stress-fat cycle with bursts of twenty-first-century adaptation of the "fight-or-flight" response.

What exercise really means for those of us over age forty is the chance to combust fat all over our bodies, especially Toxic Weight. The lovely thing about exercise is that when you find that appropriate physical activity level in addition to your appropriate nutrition and attitude, your overall health will significantly improve. Dr. Michael Pratt points out in a 1999 *Journal of the American Medical Association* editorial that the relationship between physical activity and health is very likely to be continual—meaning that some physical activity is better than none, and more is even better. If you already have problems with blood pressure and cholesterol, by dropping the first 10 percent of your body weight (at 180 pounds, this means 18 pounds), you can begin to substantially reverse the disease process just through lifestyle.

Dr. Dorian Dugmore and colleagues found in patients with heart attacks that regular, prolonged aerobic exercise improved cardiorespiratory fitness significantly. Think of exercise as training your body to be more Stress-Resilient. The benefits of physical activity translate into all other areas of your life.

Along with increased endurance for living, exercise also lowers your blood pressure. In their review of the cardiovascular benefits of exercise, Dr. William Haskell and colleagues cited several studies proving that blood pressure is lowered by aerobic exercise and that this effect is the same in people ranging in age from fifteen to eighty.

What else can exercise do for women over forty?

Exercise can

- **Reduce your risk of dying from heart disease by more than 40 percent**
- **Lower your blood pressure and cholesterol**
- **Enhance digestion and bowel regularity**
- **Shed fat by using fat more efficiently for fuel**
- **Strengthen your heart muscle**
- **Regulate your blood sugar**
- **Reduce your risk of cancer**
- **Increase strength and flexibility in joints**
- **Increase your longevity**

But the most visible result of introducing exercise into a woman's life is weight loss.

As we discussed in the Nutrition Template, physical activity is the currency with which you pay for food. I draw your attention to the Energy Balance Equation again.

The more you move, the more you can eat. It's that simple. Physical activity is actually your money in the bank. If you happen to in-

---

Figure 8-1. **Daily Energy Balance Equation**

$$\text{Total Energy Expenditure} = \text{Energy In (Food)} - \text{Energy Out (Activity)}$$

dulge in a serving of more calories than you normally eat, draw from your physical activity bank to pay for those extra calories. You don't have to panic; simply regroup and realize that you either already did extra physical activity that day to neutralize those calories or you will tomorrow. It will all balance out in the end. Your over-forty body is burning calories efficiently thanks to an exercise-induced increase in metabolic rate, and deviating from your food plan won't be cause for panic if you have gotten in your physical activity for the day.

Deb had eaten a slice of her favorite birthday cake with a scoop of ice cream. The extra 300 calories she ate were easily canceled by the extra two-mile walk she did that day (200 calories) and the rounds of golf she planned to do in the morning (200 calories). She enjoyed her birthday with none of the usual Toxic Stress of guilt. Exercise offers instant guilt relief for women like Deb who tend to be Stress Overeaters. It doesn't mean that eating the entire brownie sundae with whipped cream carries no consequence. It means you can allow yourself the occasional treat without feeling as if you have failed once again.

As you know from learning about the science of stress eating, exercise also reduces the levels of stress hormones through the release of beta-endorphins and can actually help curb your appetite for fatty foods. It's a win-win situation.

■ Questions Before We Get Started

When I explain these and other physiological effects of exercise, my patients often have questions. Here are some of the more common ones, specifically as they relate to women over the age of forty.

If you already have a known cardiovascular, pulmonary, or metabolic disease, such as diabetes, thyroid problems, renal disease, or liver disease, you must have a complete medical evaluation in order to determine the appropriate level at which you can safely exercise. This is another important element in your new self-care. The American College of Sports Medicine recommends that your medical evaluation include a symptom-limited exercise test for diagnostic purposes so you can exercise safely and effectively.

Q. How does exercise increase stamina?

A. Exercise increases your stamina or endurance, and your overall energy level. Stamina is known by exercise scientists as maximum oxygen uptake, or VO_{2max}. VO_{2max} is a fancy way of describing how efficient our bodies are at transporting oxygen and other nutrients we need to live throughout the systems of our bodies. Most exercise studies demonstrate a 10 to 20 percent increase in VO_{2max} with regular physical activity. This means that our bodies become much more efficient at transporting the oxygen and other nutrients when and where our bodies need them the most. It also means that our bodies don't have to work as hard delivering the goods. This increased "oxidative capacity" of your trained muscles, heart, and lungs also appears to have a hemodynamic effect. This means that lactic acid, a toxic byproduct that builds up in exercising muscles, decreases when we become more physically fit. (Ever "feel the burn"? That's lactic acid.) All of these wonderful adaptations to exercise result in increased stamina and endurance. This simply means that we can go longer and stronger without fatigue or muscle soreness.

Q. Why does exercise increase body strength?

A. Exercise increases your overall strength by making all of your body's internal structures (muscles, bones, tendons, ligaments, cardiovascular system, etc.) stronger. Muscles grow stronger by regularly performing activities that cause you to lift, push, or pull, such as lifting weights. If you expose your muscles to increased activity, muscles adapt by getting stronger. When you begin weight training, your muscles will adapt to this increased load by growing stronger. And stronger muscles perform more efficiently.

Training with weights stimulates your muscles to activate all the other body systems (e.g., endocrine, cardiovascular), which then adapt by growing stronger to support your stronger muscles. As your muscle fibers get stronger, the metabolic energy stores within them increase and your connective tissues (ligaments, tendons) and bones become stronger and better able to support you. All of these supporting structures are collectively known as lean body mass. Your goal is to maximize your lean body mass while at the same time decreasing your fat mass. Regular strength training increases and strengthens muscle mass, making your entire body stronger and more stressproof!

Increased muscle mass and strength are crucial for boosting your metabolism and maintaining agility as you age. Weight-bearing physical activity also leads to stronger bones, improved posture, and a decreased risk for developing osteoporosis.

Aerobic exercise causes many beneficial changes in both body and mind. When you are fit, your body is better able to deliver and use oxygen and nutrients and resist fatigue. Endurance exercise improves your overall functioning by strengthening heart and lungs, reducing levels of stress hormones circulating in your body as a result of Toxic Stress, and combusting Toxic Weight.

Q. How does exercise reduce the symptoms of menopause?

A. This is the big boy. Menopause is associated with a number of physical and emotional changes. The list of "symptoms" associated with menopause is a mile long and includes depression, weight gain, loss of muscle mass and bone density, increased risk of coronary artery disease, decrease in collagen synthesis, increase in total fat and abdominal fat mass, and increased vasomotor symptoms such as hot flashes, increased irritability, insomnia, and poor concentration. Of these symptoms, only two—vasomotor hot flashes and vaginal dryness—have been proven to be caused by hormonal changes. Exercise has not been shown to affect vaginal dryness, but it does have a demonstrated positive influence on all other negative symptoms of menopause.

Let's look at the research. One study of more than 1,600 women found that sedentary women were twice as likely to report hot flashes as physically active women. Another study reported a drop in the incidence of hot flashes immediately following a forty-five-minute aerobic workout (but not subsequently), suggesting that exercise had only an acute effect. In addition, two studies involving 267 active and sedentary women suggested that exercise-related reductions in reports of hot flashes may largely reflect the effect of exercise on mood. Most women in menopause or the perimenopause report mood disturbances. These might be related to insomnia caused by hot flashes and to neurotransmitter changes associated with aging. Studies have confirmed that regular exercise can reduce stress, whether it originates in the brain, the hormonal system (as in menopause), or the immune system.

That's not all. We now know that what most influences weight gain in the menopause is not hormonal status but the loss of muscle mass with its accompanying decrease in metabolism. Let's do the math again. Remember that for every pound of muscle lost through disuse, a woman loses the ability to burn up to 50 calories per day. Out of desperation, women resort to extreme caloric restriction to try to make up for this loss of calorie-burning metabolism. This only depresses our metabolism further.

There is hope! Exercise reverses the diet-induced reduction in metabolic rate while simultaneously increasing muscle mass. As we have already discussed, strength training is very effective in building muscles. We have definitive research showing that eight to twelve weeks of progressive weight training can substantially increase muscle strength in women aged fifty and above—even into their nineties. As I have mentioned before, do enough exercise and you will actually offset age-related changes in your body composition. Combining aerobic and weight-training exercise converts you from a weak little car into a diesel-burning 18-wheeler! You develop a more powerful engine, one that burns fuel fast and effectively.

Research has shown that you can accomplish this goal at any age. One cross-sectional study of female athletes and sedentary women aged eighteen to sixty-nine found no difference in body fat percentage and muscle mass between the youngest and oldest athletes. Additionally, the resting metabolic rate of the perimenopausal, menopausal, and postmenopausal athletes was closer to that of the young athletes than to that of the sedentary, age-matched women.

What about bone loss? Eighty percent of the twenty-five million Americans who currently have osteoporosis are women. Women's vertebral (back) and femoral (hip) bone loss usually begins after age thirty, and they can lose up to 1 percent of total bone mass yearly from age forty until menopause, when bone loss rapidly accelerates. During the first five to ten years after menopause, annual bone loss averages about 2 percent.

Without appropriate intervention a woman can easily lose up to 30 percent of her bone mass by the age of sixty. Estrogen deficiency appears to be the most important cause of bone loss. Physical activity is not a substitute for estrogen therapy for the treatment of advanced osteoporosis, but it does play a very important role. The combination of weight lifting and aerobic activity, like walking, can help prevent further bone loss and increase bone density. A study of twenty-five women aged forty-nine to sixty-one found that lumbar spine bone mineral density (BMD), which is a measure of how much bone mass is present, was significantly higher in those who jogged or played volleyball than in those who had no regular physical activity. Walking has been shown to be highly beneficial as well. A twelve-month study of more than two hundred postmenopausal women found that those who walked 7.5 miles per week had a higher average BMD of the trunk, legs, and whole body than those who walked less than one mile each week.

The risk of heart disease rises abruptly in postmenopausal women because of decreases in cholesterol and blood vessel changes induced by estrogen deficiency. You can reverse these changes by exercising. A three-year study found that the HDL cholesterol levels of healthy middle-aged women remained unchanged in those who increased their exercise over three years while it fell in those who decreased their exercise. Population studies have generally shown a strong inverse relationship between physical activity and heart disease risk and between cardiorespiratory fitness and risk of heart disease. One study of nearly fifteen hundred thirty-eight- to sixty-year-old Swedish women found that those who were the most sedentary had a nearly threefold greater incidence of coronary artery disease than those who were physically fit. An eight-year study of more than three thousand women showed that an increase in the ability to perform aerobic exercise resulted in a corresponding decrease in the risk of death from heart disease.

Q. How fast can I see results?

A. This is always the burning question as women begin their exercise programs. I have found that the rate at which you see results is based upon a number of factors. Clearly, the more time, effort, and consistency you demonstrate will hasten your results. How much muscle mass you now have determines the efficiency with which you can burn those calories. Some women are innately more athletic and comfortable with moving their bodies than others. If you have a physical disability (arthritis), then be realistic and acknowledge it will take a little longer. Here are some basic rules of the road:

■ **To remove one pound of fat from your body, you need to burn off 3,500 calories. You do that by combining healthy eating and exercise.**

- **A five-foot, four-inch woman with about fifty excess pounds can count on losing about one-half to one pound per week if, between eating well and exercising, she is burning off 250 to 500 calories per day. Walking a mile burns approximately 100 calories. The more you walk all day, the more you shed after-forty fat.**
- **You will start to see your leg muscles appear after you have been consistently (five or six times each week) accruing those forty-five minutes of aerobic activity for at least two to three months.**
- **Your menopot, as well as the Toxic Weight deep inside your abdomen, will start to decrease immediately, with belt changes noted within the first month. Some women have very efficient fat storage going on in this area of the body during perimenopause. Put some vim, vigor, and vitality into your workouts and nudge those stubborn fat cells to give up the goods!**

Whenever you have a decision to make about what to eat or whether to exercise, just remember to do the math to help you make that choice. If you eat an extra 500 calories one day, you need to pay for that somehow or it stays on your body as fat. If you exercise the next day (2.5 miles walking for a total calorie burn of 250 calories) and cut out 250 excess calories from your eating, you just neutralized the prior day's additional calories. Think like this and you become more accountable to yourself and your waistline!

Q. How will exercise affect my energy level?

A. Exercise has the amazing ability to restore your energy level, regardless of whether you suffer from fatigue or anxiety. If you are a Stress Overeater, physical activity will literally activate you, increasing your heart rate and jump-starting your day. If you are a Stress Undereater, the release of beta-endorphins will calm and soothe you. This restored energy balance will also help counter difficulty sleeping, a common problem among perimenopausal women.

The really good news is that you feel energy benefits the instant you start to exercise. After just one walk, regardless of your stress profile, you will feel a vibrant energy, an increase in hopefulness, and a decrease in sadness.

Q. Does exercise reduce the risk of heart disease?

A. Yes. The scientific literature shows a strong association between a decrease in physical activity and an increase in heart disease. There is also a clear relationship between increased regular physical activity and improvements in all of the body systems governing heart function. We have already mentioned that exercise decreases cholesterol levels, improves HDL, and reduces blood pressure. Exercise also decreases the chance of having fatal skipped heart beats, or arrhythmias. Furthermore, exercise plays a strong role in the rehabilitation of folks who have suffered a cardiac event. Data clearly indicate that patients who engage in exercise programs postevent show an increase in heart function. One study of four thousand heart patients showed that those who participated in regular exercise programs after their heart attacks had 25 percent fewer deaths from heart disease. This is a forewarning to you. Please don't wait until this happens to you to start exercising!

Q. How can exercise decrease high blood pressure?

A. Exercise reduces blood pressure by increasing the strength of the heart muscle enough to allow it to pump blood more forcefully and efficiently. The extra heart power is reflected in decreasing blood pressure measurements. People who have low levels of physical fitness have a 35 to 52 percent greater risk of developing high blood pressure. Research has also shown that regular exercise decreases blood pressure in those already diagnosed with high blood pressure.

Aerobic activity causes a temporary increase in the top (systolic) number of your blood pressure (e.g., for 120/80 blood pressure, 120 is the systolic). This increase is normal and is caused by the heart's working to increase the delivery of more blood to your working muscles. Eventually, your exercise session causes a widening of your body's blood vessels (arteries) to accommodate the increased blood flow, bringing your blood pressure back to normal again. The more physically fit you are, the more efficiently your body will normalize your blood pressure during exercise.

Q. Does exercise improve cholesterol levels?

A. Yes. Cholesterol is lowered by exercise. Cholesterol is a natural substance produced in the liver, and it is essential for helping your body build cells and in the manufacture of various hormones. When the body makes too much cholesterol, however, it, along with other fatty substances called triglycerides, causes deposits to form on the inner linings of your artery walls. These deposits are called arterial plaque. High cholesterol levels are believed to be caused by a genetic predisposition, diets high in saturated fats and cholesterol, and a sedentary lifestyle.

Exercise greatly influences how much cholesterol, primarily HDL, we have and decreases the levels of circulating triglycerides. There is a powerful negative correlation between high plasma HDL and heart disease. Endurance athletes have a 20 to 30 percent higher HDL level and lower triglyceride levels than healthy, sedentary people when compared by age.

Q. How does exercise affect my immune system?

A. The immune system's most important function, which exercise strengthens, is to defend you against cancer, infections, and other diseases. Your immune system also helps you regain health after an infectious illness or other disease. When your immune system is healthy, it can discriminate between cells that belong to you and cells that are foreign to you and must be eliminated. Aerobic exercise, such as walking briskly, stimulates your hormonal system (estrogen, progesterone, stress hormones), which in turn stimulates the immune system to become more effective. Research has shown that healthy changes in immune cell counts and function are maintained by keeping stress hormones at normal levels.

Q. How does exercise decrease risk of cancer and other diseases, such as diabetes?

A. Physical activity acts to prevent many different illnesses in so many different ways that it would be impossible for me to tell you about them all in a few simple paragraphs. The important thing to keep in mind is that exercise is vital in the prevention, as well as treatment, of many of the medical conditions that begin to emerge as we age. For instance, adult diabetes is most often associated with obesity and inactivity. Exercise increases the ability of tissues to be responsive to the body's insulin and, therefore, helps to keep blood sugars in check and diabetes under control. With proper nutrition, people with adult diabetes can often reverse the elevated blood sugars and finally get off and stay off their medicines.

Q. What is the relation between exercise and bone density gains?

A. In order for your skeleton to grow more bone (called bone modeling), it must be subjected to more weight than it is used to. Very simply, this means that the same principle I described that grows stronger muscles (the adaptation and increase in strength to respond more efficiently to regular physical challenges) also applies to your bones! Bone is actually a living tissue that is constantly changing and adapting to stresses to which it is subjected. As I have already described, some bone loss occurs naturally after age thirty and then accelerates during menopause. Results from several studies have shown that exercise minimizes bone loss by stimulating new bone growth; bones grow stronger and adapt to exercise much the same way muscles do. Studies have even shown that women in their nineties can reverse bone loss and regrow and strengthen bones with the physical stress of exercise.

I may sound like a broken record here, but once again the reduction in bone mass that has often been called "normal" with age is really due to disuse. Loss of bone, like so many other symptoms of aging, can largely be prevented by exercising regularly, quitting smoking, and making certain you get adequate nutrition (in this case, calcium).

Q. What is the relation between exercise and joint protection and resistance to injury?

A. Exercise protects your joints by strengthening the muscles surrounding them and increasing the flexibility of the tendons and ligaments that connect the joint bones to the muscles. This is a complex system of working parts in which each part actually protects the other.

The health of your skeleton depends on movement and activity. To stay healthy, your joints must do what they were made to do: move and bear weight. The health of the cartilage covering your joint surfaces is vital for maintaining proper joint function. The only way this cartilage can receive nourishment is by the manufacture and distribution of synovial fluid (think of this like motor oil lubricating moving pistons). Synovial fluid delivers nutrients, removes waste, and lubricates our joint surfaces. Movement is essential for creating this environment of joint health and for increasing the circulation of blood and lymph into and out of joint structures and the nearby soft tissues. As mammals, we were not made to sit in front of computers all day. Our bodies are marvelous machines that were made to move! If a car engine sits unused, eventually the motor oil hardens and dries up. The pistons will tighten and solidify. When you try to crank that engine up, I guarantee you will not get much power out of it. Chances are also good something will break down. Same thing with joints: if you do not move those joints, you will lose them!

Q. Can I exercise if I already have arthritis?

A. Of course! You can and should! Research studies have clearly shown improvements in both osteoarthritis and rheumatoid arthritis with walking and strengthening exercises. These improvements include decreased pain and increased range of motion.

Q. What is the relationship between exercise and depression?

A. As we have already noted, exercise is equally, if not more, effective than traditional antidepressants for mild to moderate depression. The beta-endorphin that is secreted during exercise is a powerful modulator of mood and can help increase hopefulness and permit better clarity of thinking and focus, instead of despair and frustration. I am not suggesting exercise in place of other therapies, but your doctor may decide to reevaluate certain medications once you begin exercising regularly.

■ Money in the Bank

Now that you know the endless benefits of physical activity, specifically, what do I recommend? After the age of forty, exercise becomes a nonnegotiable part of everyday life. Your goal is to accrue at least forty-five minutes of some form of aerobic physical activity at least five or six times per week. Then twice per week, in addition to your aerobic activity, add at least thirty minutes of strength training.

The idea of accruing exercise is important because many women simply don't have a block of time every morning or evening to fit in a workout. But you might have fifteen minutes in the morning, fifteen minutes at lunch, and another fifteen minutes sometime in the afternoon or evening. And, naturally, each day is different. But accruing exercise throughout the day is just as beneficial as taking one forty-five-minute exercise class. This is similar to my recommendation that you drink eight glasses of water daily. I don't expect you to gulp down all eight glasses at one sitting. *Accruing* forty-five minutes of physical activity each day is possible, even for the busiest woman.

Spreading your activity throughout the day can act like sustained release energy boosters as well as stress neutralizers. Many women who can get in their forty-five minutes all at one time still stay as active as they can throughout the day, constantly adding more currency to their physical activity bank. It really is like money in the bank. One of my patients, Jane, gave me a piggy bank she had painted. On its side were listed all the ways she accrues exercise: walking at lunch, climbing the stairs on a coffee break, walking to and from the bus stop and subway, and on and on. The concept of accrual is an opportunity to find creative ways to meet *your needs*.

I'm not talking about tae bo, kickboxing at dawn, or running thirty miles every week in the sleet and snow. You don't need to join the Olympics. Exercise, for the over-forty woman, can be as fun and simple as a brisk walk outside or on a treadmill, biking, swimming, or lifting light weights. Dancing, aerobics, Jazzercise, tennis, cross-country skiing, golf, and hiking are also excellent (and social) forms of exercise. Many women have also taken up rowing in recent years.

The trick is to find something that's fun for you to do, something that you look forward to doing. And remember that all of this will continually be refined and redone the rest of your life. As each year passes, you may want to experiment and try new things. I happen to love mountain climbing, but it's not a very practical daily sport, so I take long, enjoyable walks instead and daydream about a spring trip out west. I also love to take "walk and talks" with my patients. For these sessions, we put on our sneakers and walk about the picturesque neighborhood surrounding my office instead of sitting inside for our appointment.

Okay, I'm a realist. It's probably because I am a doctor—not a so-called fitness expert—and I have seen so many patients over the years. The point is to do something physical every day that will not only help reduce stress but will also keep your body toned and fit.

Our over-forty exercise goes beyond our need for aerobic exercise. While the grand majority of perimenopausal women have not been exposed to any formal strength training, it's not too late. My first caveat is this: women are much stronger than they think. It's not about muscles; it's about strength. And I know you are capable.

When your child darted out from between parked cars, how fast did you run to stop her? How many times did you carry the groceries from the store to the car and then from the car to the kitchen?

You are strong. You do have the potential. And I'm serious about your needing to get started with strength training. Research now shows that women who do not strength train lose at least seven pounds of muscle every ten years. Although Jazzercise or walking improves cardiovascular fitness, they do not prevent the loss of muscle tissue. As you just learned, building muscle mass and strength is vital to combating natural and diet-induced metabolic decreases and to increasing bone density, balance, and agility.

When they first come to me, many of my patients are dissociated from their bodies, meaning their bodies seem foreign and separate. We need to reassociate. Physical activity connects our minds and bodies. One of the most lasting results is that as a woman becomes physically stronger, she also becomes mentally stronger. Self-esteem, for any women over forty, must now begin to come from physical as well as mental achievement. It must spring from a deep commitment to self-care, something women of our generation have not been very good at. Not a once-a-week massage or manicure. I'm talking about *a concentrated effort to put your needs first.*

You need to eliminate chronic Toxic Stress from

■ **Relationships**
■ **Eating**
■ **Physical activity**

For women over forty, the three nonnegotiable aspects of the Physical Activity Template are:

1. **Accruing forty-five minutes of exercise five or six days a week;**
2. **Beginning whole body strength training at least twice per week;**
3. **Performing stretches every day.**

Think about how you can incorporate your need for stress-neutralizing physical activity into Plan A and Plan B. Remember to calm down and simply formulate a different and workable plan if your normal routine is upset. Your gym is closed today for renovation? Take that walk outdoors instead.

Try to get in your exercise at a time when you will be least likely to be interrupted. Many women prefer including some physical activity during the morning hours before their busy day makes it tough to get it in. For the Stress Undereater who wakes up agitated and ill at ease, this morning activity will start the day off right by decreasing the amount of Alarm Hormone circulating in the body. Stress Overeaters, on the other hand, will benefit from the activating properties of exercise and feel more alert and ready to face the day.

When it comes to physical activity, KISS. Even if you're really fit, walking is great exercise. It's good for building bone density because it's weight bearing; it's easy for most people; it doesn't require a lot of fancy equipment; it can be done almost anywhere; it burns calories; it improves heart health; and it is stress reducing.

Even if you've always done some other sort of aerobic exercise, I want you to try to incorporate more walking into your day. It's one of the things we can do to add little deposits of money in the bank throughout the day, stoking our metabolic furnace fires and helping us efficiently burn up our calories and that over-forty fat. Whether you are walking on a treadmill or walking on the moon, you need a minimum of forty-five minutes of aerobic physical activity *five or six days a week*. This forty-five-minute period may be broken up for convenience without decreasing its benefit. The American College of Sports Medicine confirms that physical activity can be accumulated in short periods, such as ten minutes, throughout the day. Aerobic fitness is the foundation of your destressing exercise program.

But remember that aerobic exercise is just one of the necessary components of your over-forty exercise plan. The second component is strength training, which becomes more important as we age as it ensures that we'll maintain agility, balance, and self-sufficiency, as well as boost our metabolism. Flexibility is the third, and frequently neglected, component of exercise. This refers to how far your muscles can extend, how elastic they are. Flexibility is needed for balance and agility, particularly to avoid falls as we age and to help you perform a variety of physical functions.

I will expand on the concepts of strength training and flexibility in the next chapter, but I want you to keep in mind that regular exercise involves these in addition to your aerobic activity.

■ Tools to Get Started

Before starting your aerobic exercise program, we need to see how strong your heart and lungs are. Don't worry; they are probably stronger than you think!

We need to know what your resting heart rate is in order to determine your beginning fitness level. As you continue to be more physically active, your resting heart rate will decrease, indicating that your heart muscle is getting stronger and more efficient at pumping blood throughout your body. Monitoring your heart rate is a great way to get *feedback from your body* as you progress. Your body is saying "Thanks!" for allowing it to perform optimally.

All women over forty should first have a complete medical evaluation to determine the safe and appropriate level of exercise to begin with. If you are a woman at risk for or have already been diagnosed with any medical condition, including heart or thyroid disease, diabetes, or any metabolic disorder, it is imperative that you exercise under the careful supervision of your doctor. The American College of Sports Medicine recommends that your medical evaluation include a physical activity stress test to determine whether you may have any underlying medical problems, so that you can exercise safely and effectively.

Work Sheet I: The Heart Check

1. To perform the Heart Check, you will need: a pair of supportive sneakers; comfortable clothes; a watch or clock with a second hand, or a stopwatch; a measured mile on flat terrain or a sturdy treadmill.

2. Go to the start of your measured mile and warm up for two minutes by walking slowly, swinging your arms and lifting your knees high. Rest for another two minutes.

3. At the start of your measured mile, note the time on the chart below.

4. Walk the mile as fast as you can.

5. If you can't finish the mile, note your distance, time, and pulse for future comparison.

6. If you do finish, note the time on the chart below.

7. Immediately take your pulse and note that too.

Starting time: _____

Ending time: _____

Walking time: _____

Walking time (rounded to the nearest whole minute): _____

Ending pulse: _____

Distance walked: _____ (one mile unless unable to complete distance).

Now refer to the Rockport Fitness Walking Test charts in Appendix C to determine your level. Locate the appropriate one for your age. Along the bottom of this chart, find the time it took you to walk the mile and draw a vertical line up from that point. Along the side of this chart, find your pulse (taken after the completion of the mile) and draw a horizontal line from that point. Read your fitness level at the point where the lines cross.

Results:

Unable to complete the mile	Level 1
Scored in "low" or "below average"	Level 1
Scored in "average"	Level 2
Scored in "above average" or "high"	Level 3

Heart Check Level: _____

Work Sheet 2: Taking Your Pulse

Your pulse tells you how hard your heart is working. Before taking your pulse, read the Heart Check (see page 209).

1. To take your pulse, you will need a watch or clock with a second hand or a stopwatch.

2. Place the first two fingers of one hand (never the thumb, which has its own pulse) on the wrist of the other, just below your thumb. Feel around until you find a pulse.

3. If you can't find your pulse at your wrist, find the carotid artery in your neck. With the same two fingers, feel up under your jawbone about halfway between your ear and your chin. Be careful, though; some people are at risk for fainting when they compress the carotid artery, so don't press too hard!

4. Using a second hand on a clock or watch or a stopwatch, count the number of beats for fifteen seconds and write the number below.

5. Count it again to double-check.

6. Multiply the number by 4 to get your pulse.

15-second pulse: _____

15-second pulse (second try): _____

1-minute pulse (15-second pulse x 4): _____

■ Workout Schedule

Level 1: You have probably never been involved in regular physical activity before. Wait one day between completing the assessment and starting your workout to give your body time to recover. I want you to start with thirty-minute walks at a comfortable pace, or two fifteen-minute walks, going as fast as you can while still being able to carry on a conversation. Wait one day between walks.

Level 2: You are in good shape but need to reintroduce *regular* exercise into your life. Begin with forty minutes at a brisk pace and maybe power-walk up a few hills. Walk every other day. Gradually increase this to walking five or six days a week, and then add five minutes to your walks.

Level 3: You are in very good shape. Let's continue that trend! Start by walking for forty-five minutes as fast as you can. Go up hills whenever you find them. Walk four to seven days a week. Build up to fifty minutes to an hour, every day, as you get fitter. Do the walk in addition to any workouts you were already doing.

Changing levels: In two to three months, you'll probably be ready for a change. Your walks will have gotten too easy—and maybe a little boring. One day, instead of your walk, do the one-mile test again to see if you've made it to the next level. If so, go for that workout. If not, pick an amount in between the two levels and do that until you make it to the next level.

■ Exercise Intensity

Ideally, the aerobic activity you choose must work the large muscle groups in your legs, arms, back, and abdomen. The activity should be done in a continual, rhythmic manner, and it must be capable of elevating your heart rate to 60 to 90 percent of your age-predicted maximum; your age-predicted maximum heart rate is 220 minus your age. These physiological changes will not occur during window-shopping, doubles tennis, or while you are walking the dog around the block.

Here is an example: Strolling around the mall, you spend the entire afternoon on your feet. You wander out to the car and are amazed to realize you just spent three hours walking and standing—you never sat down at all. Another day, you push the lawn mower around. After half an hour, it's time for a cool drink and a lounge chair. You're sweating; your heart is beating away. That's intensity.

One way to monitor your level of intensity is to use something exercise scientists call the rate of perceived exertion scale. This helps you to know what your level of exertion or intensity is as you perform physical activity. On a scale of zero to ten, sleeping is a zero, shopping is a two, and moving the lawn mower for half an hour is about a five. Here are some other examples to help you determine your actual rate of exertion.

Women who spend more time more intensely active will be better prepared to run after children—or tennis balls or buses! As you go through each day, ask yourself at which end of the scale did you

Table 8-1. **Rate of Perceived Exertion**

Rating	Perceived Exertion	Examples of Exertion
0	nothing at all	sleeping
1	very, very weak	lying on the couch watching TV, reading a book, going to the movies, attending a meeting at work
2	weak	shopping, sitting at dinner, playing the piano, doing the laundry, sitting at your desk
3	moderate	walking the dog, playing doubles tennis, walking to work
4	somewhat strong	gardening, climbing hills, cycling for pleasure
5	strong, somewhat hard	walking very fast, you are still able to talk but not to sing; mowing the lawn
6	fairly strong, hard	walking very, very fast; it is uncomfortable but you are able to do it
7	very strong, feels hard and you don't think you can carry this on for very long	running fairly fast, chopping wood, lifting very heavy weights, cross-country skiing
8	very, very strong, must force yourself to do this	running as fast as you can, jumping rope, kickboxing without stopping
9	very, very hard	running in the Olympics
10	very, very hard; maximal	running for your life

spend most of your time and how can you get more active throughout your twenty-four hours of living.

That brings me back to your aerobics workouts. For the most benefit, you should work at an intensity level of between six and seven during your aerobic physical activity. Yes, you should be able to carry on a conversation (but not a very chatty one!).

Fat-Burning Workouts

Higher intensity workouts are more efficient at burning fat. Research shows that you burn more calories from harder work, and you get to do it in less time.

Intense fat-burning workouts at high intensity not only help you shed your over-forty fat, but they also let you blow off chronic Toxic Stress. They will get your heart pumping and muscles exercising while you bring your stress hormones back to normal levels. Sweaty workouts are 100 percent guaranteed to produce a sense of control and calm in your life. They help you to become more Stress-Resilient throughout the day.

If, on the other hand, you need some peace and the idea of a tough workout is making you cringe, go for the slower, softer kind. There's nothing wrong at all with interspersing less intense workouts with more vigorous ones. We have all had tough days when just getting up and finding your gym shoes is the real challenge. Don't worry. Just move anyway. Go for a stroll, stop to look at the leaves, and save the pavement pounding for tomorrow.

So, walking briskly at a rate of about 3.5 to 4 miles per hour will provide the desired intensity. Walking thirty minutes at a very, very vigorous pace is equivalent to running two miles! Whatever activity you choose, aerobic training means increasing your body's demand for oxygen and maintaining that demand for a certain amount of time. While you do not have to run a marathon (although you may want to walk one someday, as some of my patients have done), the exercise must be intense enough to cause your heart and lungs to work harder than usual. Remember to put gusto into those steps!

Don't run from vigor in your activities. It's really good for you. Think of yourself as an expensive, powerful sports car. It needs to be taken our regularly for a drive at high speed to keep it functioning optimally. This is the same for that marvelous body of yours. You need to challenge it with vigor and gusto to keep it operating to the best of its ability.

Once you get your basic fitness down, you can alter your routine to spice it up a little. Alternate days of long duration with lighter days. Devote particular days to increasing strength or speed. You can use another activity one or two days per week to cross-train and work your muscles in different ways.

■ Other Aerobic Workouts

I'm certainly not going to restrict you to walking, even though it's so great. If you like to cycle, take step classes, or jog, more power to you. As you progress through the levels, you'll want your goal to be at least five or six workouts every week that really work your heart. The following workouts are all good options for building heart fitness, and stamina. Most of them also have other benefits, which are on the chart too. For some of these activities, the pace is specified. For others, shoot for that six or seven in intensity. The calories are calculated for a 150-pound woman working out for thirty minutes. If you weigh more, you'll burn more and vice versa.

Every woman is uniquely endowed with a body that may be more appropriate for engaging in a particular physical activity. My tall stature made me great for volleyball and basketball, but a royal klutz in gymnastics. Take a moment and assess your individual attributes. Innately strong upper bodies make powerful rowers and swimmers. Sturdy legs make hiking, climbing, and biking possible. Remember, life's an adventure! Experiment, challenge yourself, have fun, and see which physical activities work for you. The bottom line is *for you to get up and move* that wonderful body of yours every day you can!

Table 8-2. **Aerobic Workouts**

Workout	Calories Burned	Other Significant Benefits
(based on a 150-pound woman working out for 30 minutes)		
Aerobics class, easy	210	leg strength, flexibility, bone density
Aerobics class, hard	276	leg strength, flexibility, bone density
Ballroom dancing	105	leg strength, balance

Cross-country skiing	231	leg, torso, and arm strength, balance and coordination
Cycling (at 5.5 mph)	132	leg strength
Cycling (at 9.4 mph)	204	leg strength
Golf (no cart)	174	torso strength, leg strength, upper-body flexibility
Ice skating	192	leg strength, balance and coordination
In-line skating	192	leg and torso strength, balance and coordination
Jumping rope (70 jumps per min.)	330	bone density, leg strength, coordination
Marching in place, fast	291	leg strength, bone density
Racquetball	363	speed, flexibility, bone density, overall strength
Running (11.5 min/mi)	276	leg strength, bone density
Running (9 min/mi)	393	leg strength, bone density
Skiing, green trails	243	leg strength, balance, and coordination
Snowshoeing, soft snow	339	leg strength, balance
Stair climbing	206	leg strength, bone density
Swimming, slow crawl	261	flexibility, overall strength
Swimming, fast crawl	318	flexibility, overall strength
Tennis, moderate singles	222	leg strength, bone density, flexibility, some torso and arm strength, coordination
Uphill hiking	246	leg strength, bone density
Walking (at 6 mph)	260	leg strength and bone density

■ Exercise Expectations

Right now, you probably think that exercise is like dieting. You do it for a week or two because you're supposed to, you stress over missed workouts, you hop on the scale to see results. Then something interrupts your schedule; you miss a few days. You get wrapped up in the other pressures of life and, before you know it, months have passed since you last put on your sneakers.

Exercise is not about trudging to your workout, getting sore muscles, rushing around the gym. It's about moving your body every day, easing the transition through menopause and leading a healthy, balanced, enjoyable life. And honoring the really important priorities in your life. Your family and friends are the genuine treasures in life. You, in turn, are their greatest gift. Take care of your gift to them by acknowledging that your body needs care and attention. If you neglect yourself, if you don't exercise, if you continue to eat self-destructively, you will not only shorten your life, but you will also bring sadness to your loved ones.

Imagine the pages of a family album. Now mentally flip through to the end. Graduations. Weddings. Grandchildren. Golden anniversaries. Don't voluntarily take yourself out of those pictures prematurely. Make the commitment now to be there for the ones you love and those who love you.

Let's talk expectations. First, what do you expect in return for doing your daily physical activity? Make a list of all the things you expect:

1.
2.
3.
4.
5.

For some of my patients, the list may include "more energy," "more stamina," "fitting better into clothes," "lessened anxiety." Each woman is unique and every situation different. Every journey starts with a first step. The moment you put on your sneakers, you have begun.

Second, you must decide how much time and effort you are willing to give this. I call this learning how to "price" your self-care. If you have decided to spend a very little amount of time exercising and attending to healthy eating, you have paid a small price. You will feel and look like it. Conversely, women who can routinely find the baseline amount of time to care for their bodies feel and appear more energetic, vibrant, and centered, and they look fit and terrific! Pay the price and reap the rewards.

Third, be patient with yourself. You didn't achieve your career goals or raise your children overnight; you are not going to become physically fit over night. Each activity involves a lifetime commitment. Every day you can realistically say "I am getting stronger. It is easier to hold on to a healthy weight." Every day you can tell yourself "I am building stronger muscles. I am removing and combusting excess Toxic Weight, and I feel great." Instant results are a myth.

Women often expect to change overnight, and the media has led them to believe this transformation is quick and easy. But our bodies are complex biological systems. Nothing meaningful or sustainable is accomplished with shortcuts and quick fixes. These false cures just create more Toxic Stress. How long it takes before you see a difference depends upon where you are starting from and what price you are willing to pay. If you want it enough that you are working out steadily every day, including vigorous weight training twice a week, you will see results sooner. But you need to be patient with the changes.

Finally, remember to stay realistic and practice your regrouping. Acknowledge every day that your best laid Plan A routines will be constantly challenged every hour by your busy life. *Learn to expect these interruptions.* Be prepared to switch to a Plan B routine whenever you need to, and simply do the best you can to tread weight.

When my patient Gioia was away for a week at an intense business conference, her Plan B involved using the hotel fitness room when she could, taking walks outside, or using the stairs instead of the elevators or escalators. She would rather have been home on her own treadmill but she adjusted to her circumstances. Sometimes a day would go by with no opportunity to do any of these things. No big deal. Gioia simply adjusted her eating based upon limited activity and got back to her Plan A routine when she finally returned home. Gioia demonstrates, once again, that health results from the successful adaptation to life's stresses.

■ Finding the Place and Time to Make Fitness Possible

Just as work and social plans go into your date book so you don't forget them, make appointments with yourself to work out. Be courageous and write your workout times in *pen*. Briefly describe your workouts in a journal. Take a moment and simply write down the time you spent working out and what you accomplished. For example, "45 minutes stationary bike," or "pretty autumn morning; had fun walking in the neighborhood with Amy, 35 minutes, 2 miles." It takes less than a minute to write. Why do this? These descriptions give us valuable feedback about how we are learning to care for ourselves.

Looking back on the pages after a month, you can see the patterns of your activities. They say so much about how we live and prioritize our time. You can observe your own creativity in getting in time for yourself. At the same time, you can clearly see the struggle it often involves to fight for the little time it takes to care for your body. In essence, you see yourself cope and adapt.

Giving yourself a sacred space is one of the first steps. By "space" I mean both the place and the time. You deserve it and you can make it happen. You deserve a piece of floor where you can stretch away the tension of the day. You have earned a comfortable chair, a decent treadmill, good sneakers, and whatever else you need. These are yours.

I want you to choose an environment to exercise in that is not psychologically stressful. Many women may find a gym environment to be particularly distressing. Surrounded by women swathed in Spandex and thonged leotards, the over-forty woman can feel intimidated, depressed, and distracted from carrying out her own exercise routine. If you'd rather work out at home or elsewhere with friends—great! Walking on your treadmill or in your neighborhood, or seeing a trainer at home works for many of my patients. The key is to make your exercise routine as stress reducing as possible. Choose a sacred space that makes this happen for you.

So, let's think specifically about how you can begin to integrate physical activity into your day to neutralize stress and stress eating. First, let's look at the issue of timing of the workouts.

Plan to exercise appropriately around mealtime. You can exercise right before eating a main meal. You will then have a healthy appetite and burn your calories efficiently. Or you can exercise about one to one and a half hours after the main meal. That is because you must allow your digestive hormones, especially insulin, to go back to their normal levels to allow you to use your fat and carbohydrate body fuel optimally. Of course, you can take a nice walk after any meal. It's just that you cannot become vigorous or use your fat stores well right after a meal. Please continue to do the after-dinner stroll, as it will obviously use some calories and is enjoyable. Just schedule another time to do the more intense, fat-burning workout.

Also, it's fine to have a small snack before your vigorous workout if you are truly hungry. Examples include a small banana, an apple, or a piece of toast. It's silly to starve through a workout when all you need is a little High-Quality/Low-Stress energy boost. This small amount of food will not interfere with your fat burning.

Second, as I have already mentioned, be realistic and plan to exercise at a time when you'll be least bothered and interrupted by others.

Next, remember to time it so that you can let your stress hormone biorhythm work best for you. Using trial and error, find out which part of your daily biorhythm optimizes your exercise enjoyment and effectiveness. Remember that every time you get up and move your body, if even for just a minute or two, you increase your energy level instantly, regardless of time of day. This is especially important as you enter the CortiZone each day, when your energy, focus, and concentration are really beginning to dip, and fatigue and mindlessness begin to set in.

For example, some women find that in the morning, as stress hormones are peaking, their level of focus and energy is greatest, and the chance of interruption is lowest. Others may find that the energy boost they get from having a workout at lunchtime, in the midafternoon, or after work helps to counter the declining energy they feel as stress hormone levels drop off. Optimally, your goal is to get in that forty-five minutes of aerobic activity at once or accrued throughout the day, and then add to that whatever physical movements you can do additionally (getting up from your desk and moving around for three minutes after sitting at your computer for one hour).

Finally, a word about fatigue. As many people enter the CortiZone time of day, they naturally begin to feel the fatigue that is brought on by declining stress hormone levels. Stress and frustration levels are climbing and they are feeling tired and unfocused. The biggest mistake they make is to think that eating a Low-Quality/High-Stress food—a vending machine cookie or candy—will energize them. As we have already pointed out, it only makes things worse. Instead, the optimal way to deal with this is to first eat a midafternoon snack of High-Quality/Low-Stress foods, as we have described in the Nutrition Template. Then combine this with getting up and moving around for at least three to five minutes or more. Either of these activities, and especially in combination, will energize and refocus you so that you can finish your day without self-destructive eating.

My patient Barbara once noted that when you're wishing you could catch a quick nap in the middle of a busy and stressful day, go for a brisk ten-minute walk. It's like magic. It gets your blood flowing and makes the rest of the day brighter.

My patients have a variety of additional suggestions for keeping

---

Table 8-3. **Daily Stress Hormone Management: Aerobic Activity Plans**

Getting in the Baseline Aerobic Activity by Working Around Meals

1. 45 minutes before breakfast, lunch, midafternoon snack, or dinner
2. 1.5 hours after breakfast, lunch, or dinner
3. 30 to 45 minutes after the midafternoon snack
4. 10- or 15-minute increments divided throughout the day, before or 1.5 hours after meals

Getting More Energy from Extra Activity

1. Using stairs, getting up, stretching, and moving around for 3 to 5 minutes as often as possible throughout the day

Navigating the CortiZone

1. As energy dips starting around 3 P.M., get up and move as frequently as you can for at least 3 to 5 minutes to boost energy and regain focus
2. Never forget your midafternoon snack

on track with their stress-neutralizing activity. Jean emphasizes the importance of having a schedule. She puts her exercise routine as the first thing in her day. "When that is done, the hardest part of my day is over." Deb notes that a social support system is absolutely critical. Deb's husband joins her on her daily three-milk walk. Like Deb, ask your husband and children to join you, or come up with simultaneous workouts—jog around the field when the kids are at soccer or baseball practice. Instead of driving to the store or restaurant for dinner, ask your husband to walk with you. Johari and Naomi have time-saving tricks that may also encourage you to get to your morning exercise. Johari lays out exercise clothes for herself in the evening so they are readily available while Naomi sleeps in hers, so all she has to do before exercising in the morning is put on her sneakers.

■ Getting Prepared for Moving Your Body

In the next chapter, we'll get you ready for some simple but necessary strength training with exercises you can do anywhere. But before you begin either the aerobic workout or the ones that follow in Chapter 9, give your doctor a call to double-check that there's no reason you need to take extra precautions, especially if you've been sedentary. One of the reasons people stop exercising despite great New Year's resolutions is that they overdo it in the beginning. Be patient and listen to your body. Start this exercise journey with care and caution as you awaken your muscles and joints and take those first steps. Yes, you'll shed that over-forty weight, but try to go beyond just weight loss as the focus. Feel the energy replace the stress as you begin to move your body. After years of Toxic Stress and dissociation, your mind and body are a team reunited to keep you healthy and fit.

9 To Remove Weight You Have to Lift Weight

By now you know how important it is to get up and move your body aerobically. In this chapter we're going to look at the second and third critical components of your over-forty exercise needs: strength training, or weight lifting, and flexibility.

Many women, perhaps a majority, often believe that doing some form of regular aerobic exercise is all they need to stay fit and strong for the rest of their lives. We now know that weight lifting *in combination* with aerobic exercise is a nonnegotiable essential in every over-forty woman's life. Actually, it is the secret to success to removing weight as well as to keeping it off.

- Muscles: Your Calorie-Burning Furnace

- The KISS (Keep It Sublimely Simple) Home Workout Plan: How to Stretch and Lift Weight Safely so You Can Remove Weight

- Stress Profile Exercise Prescriptions

Researchers at the University of Pittsburgh and the Colorado Health Sciences Center have compiled a national weight control registry of more than 2,800 men and women who have lost at least 30 pounds and kept them off for five to ten years. How did they do it? By burning calories through exercise every day that they could. The numbers are extraordinary. Each of these men and women burned more than 2,800 calories per week, or about 400 calories daily, with exercise. Remember that a walk burns 100 calories, and walking was the most popular mode of aerobic exercise, accounting for 1,000 calories per week of caloric burn.

The other weekly 1,800 calories were burned up in cross-training with other forms of aerobic activities such as biking. The clincher is that the majority of the registry participants engaged in some form of strength training. Aerobic activity alone is not enough. You need to lift weights.

■ Muscles: Your Calorie-Burning Furnace

I often hear from women that they are intimidated by the thought of lifting weights. "I've never strength trained before," they tell me. Any woman who is currently in her forties or fifties was rarely taught to lift weights in a PE class. Even many female athletes did not formally incorporate weight lifting into their training until the 1980s. With so little exposure to this training, why should we feel naturally inclined today to go to a gym to work out or to lift dumbbells in our living rooms?

The truth is, you *have* lifted weights. You might not have called it strength training, but what do you think quickly lifting your thirty-five-pound son or daughter away from that hot oven is? You have spent years hoisting children and packing boxes, book bags, briefcases, and grocery bags—all of these are much heavier than my beginning weight workouts. Women need to be reminded that they are innately strong.

Muscular strength is so important because it is one of the primary factors involved in boosting your midlife metabolism. As you learned in the last chapter, muscles are like a furnace: They help you burn more calories even when at rest and help you stay metabolically warmer. Because muscle is so metabolically active, any loss of muscle tissue reduces our resting metabolic rate. Without regular strength training to build and maintain muscle mass, your body's metabolism cools down over time and burns fewer and fewer calories. According to a 1992 study, women who do not strength train lose about 7 pounds of muscle every ten years and experience a reduction in metabolism equal to at least 350 calories per day. Of great interest is another study of sixty-five women that reported that *the age-related decline in resting metabolic rate is not observed in women who participate in regular exercise.* Aerobic exercise improves cardiovascular fitness, but it does not keep us from losing muscle tissue. Simply stated, strength training with weights increases muscle mass and decreases fat. Let's look at some reality checks about women and their muscles.

Changes in your muscles are related to reductions in a number of factors. Between the ages of thirty and eighty, the overall strength of your back, arm, and leg muscles can drop as much as 60 percent. This largely reflects a progressive loss of muscle mass at an average rate of 4 percent per decade from ages twenty-five to fifty, and 10 percent per decade thereafter. Along with age-related changes, reduced fitness level is the primary culprit of this decrease in strength. Muscular endurance declines as well, leading to more rapid fatigue. Studies of animals have found that the muscles' ability to provide sustained power during contraction diminishes by up to 50 percent with age. Aging muscles are also more easily injured and take longer to recover. This increased vulnerability can be profound but can also be extremely important—and not in a good way. Protracted healing lengthens the period of immobility due to pain; if this period is long enough, normal strength may never return. Newly weakened muscle will be further vulnerable to future injury. Once set in motion, this vicious cycle of frailty is very difficult to interrupt. Now the good news.

There is also a growing body of research evidence which shows that exercising at a sufficient intensity can increase strength in your muscles just as effectively as in younger individuals. Most heartening of all is research documenting the substantial benefits of training with weights, even into the tenth decade of life. One study enrolled ten frail nursing home residents, aged eighty-six to ninety-six, in eight weeks of high-intensity weight-lifting exercise. For the nine who completed the study, the quadriceps (thigh muscle) strength increased progressively, to a mean of 74 percent above baseline strength at the program's end. Midthigh muscle area also increased. Most important, significant functional improvements accompanied these strength and muscle mass gains. In five of the subjects who were assessed, gait speed increased by nearly 50 percent, and two of the subjects no longer needed canes to walk.

The bottom line is that it's never too late to improve your muscles. One of my most successful patients is an elegant seventy-two-year-old woman who, after incorporating aerobic and strength training into her life, decreased her menopot enough to drop two dress sizes with a weight loss of 15 pounds. Adding weight lifting to your life makes you fit into your clothes better and quicker than if you only did aerobic exercise. Weight lifting shapes you like nothing else.

Study after study shows that women over forty *can and should* participate in strength training and, furthermore, that they will reap tremendous proven scientific benefits. A 1995 study of fifteen postmenopausal women found that weight training increased muscle mass and resting metabolic rate along with weight loss. It also showed that strength increased in various muscle groups anywhere from 20 to 190 percent! Another study of twenty-one women ages sixty to seventy-five years showed that women who participated in twelve weeks of aerobic exercise and strength training had twice the stamina as those women who participated only in the aerobic training.

■ How We Build Strength

How does a woman actually increase her strength by weight lifting? The answer lies in how your muscles function. Each muscle in your body is a bundle of fibers running in a particular direction. Each of these fibers is comprised of a group of muscle cells. When you pick up a 5-pound weight to do a biceps curl, your nervous system sends a signal to these cells to contract, or shorten, the muscles in the front of your upper arms. In response to the signal, changes in protein strands in each muscle cell cause the muscle as a whole to contract. When you complete the movement by lowering the weight back to the starting position, your muscles return to their original, relaxed and lengthened, state.

■ Why Mild Muscle Soreness Is a Good Thing

There are two kinds of activity-related muscle soreness. The first is soreness that occurs immediately after you exercise. This usually reflects simple fatigue caused by a buildup in your muscles of the biochemical waste products of exercise (remember lactic acid from Chapter 8?). This burning discomfort normally subsides after a minute or two of rest, after which you can resume your exercise, almost always without any residual side effects. If discomfort persists after the rest, you should stop the activity and rest the part of your body that is involved.

The second type of soreness is called delayed-onset muscle soreness (DOMS) and usually develops within a day or two of exercising (at least twelve hours after). DOMS after a workout is common, especially when you first begin exercising or while you are shifting levels. You will often be most sore the first two days after beginning your workouts. It's okay! It simply means your body is not used to the activity. You may also notice some muscle stiffness and weakness. These feelings are a normal response and are part of an adaptation process that leads to greater strength once the muscles recover.

If you challenge your body *regularly* by lifting something you aren't used to (like a dumbbell weight) or you lift something that is heavier than your body is accustomed to (a heavy child), the muscles involved become stronger as a result. This happens because the active muscles develop microscopic tears in them. Your wonderfully adaptive body responds to these tears by producing new muscle fibers to rebuild itself. These repaired fibers heal stronger, and the newly added muscle fibers increase your overall muscle mass.

The amount of microscopic tearing in your muscles depends on how hard and how long you exercise and what types of exercise you are doing. For example, activities in which your muscles forcefully contract at the same time as they are lengthening tend to cause the most soreness. These "eccentric" contractions serve as brakes in activities such as running down stairs, running downhill, lowering weights, and performing the downward movements in the squats and push-ups included later in this chapter.

In addition to this microscopic tearing, swelling may take place in and around your muscles, which can also contribute to delayed soreness. This mild swelling increases pressure on the neighboring structures of joints, ligaments, and tendons, resulting in feelings of stiffness. Don't be discouraged, though—mild soreness after a workout is a sign that your muscles are healing stronger and firmer than before! That is exactly the goal for which you are aiming: new muscle fibers growing while slightly damaged muscles rebuild. This is how your muscles become larger and increase strength. This rebuilding process is why it is important to take a day off between strength-training workouts; you need to give your muscles at least twenty-four hours to repair. Think of this as your muscles' way of regrouping. The muscles are strengthening and adapting to handle the new "stress" of strength training!

If the soreness is really a problem, you can do things to help minimize this condition. One very important step is to warm up and stretch thoroughly before every activity and cool down completely afterward. This is done by performing some rhythmic movement for about three to five minutes and then gently stretching the muscles. It's also important to give your muscles time to adapt to your new activity. Don't try to do too much too soon. If you have been inactive and your goal is to walk three miles in forty-five minutes, begin by walking a mile, then add another quarter mile at each workout until you can comfortably walk three miles. Once you reach the distance goal of comfortably walking three miles, then you can pick up the pace and increase your walking speed to achieve your goal of three miles in forty-five minutes.

Be gentle with yourself and you will do just fine! You should allow any soreness or stiffness to thoroughly subside before exercising the affected muscles again, making sure to warm up and stretch. If the pain is sharp or persists longer than seven days, consult your physician.

■ A Quick Note About Muscle Building

For most of you who have never done strength-training workouts, let me assure you that you will not end up looking like a contestant in a bodybuilding contest. There is a very small minority of women who are genetically endowed with a larger muscle mass. Unless you are one of these rare individuals, you need not worry about developing bulky muscles. In reality, most women who strength-train regularly develop a lovely curvaceous and fit body.

Naomi, a Stress Overeater who runs her own marketing research company, began weight training at the age of fifty-two, when she first became my patient. Hesitant at first, she was surprised by the results:

"I actually have cleavage for the first time in my life." Her cup size increased because she built up the pectoral muscles under her breasts. Her pants fit better at a higher weight than she had expected. Naomi's strength training provides her with physical benefits that make her busy life easier. For instance, in her current workout, she bench presses 60 pounds every week, which keeps her from straining and hurting her shoulder when she hoists her 45-pound bag into the overhead compartment in planes three days a week.

Naomi works hard at her strength training. She gets sore afterward, but not as sore as she used to get from constant shoulder injuries. She feels stronger in general. This is what I want for you.

A 1993 research review concluded that maintaining body strength is integral to maintaining functional ability and self-sufficiency and to preventing falls in old age. We must recognize our *need* for strength training to maintain health during the second half of our lives.

■ Tools to Get Started

First we need to evaluate your current condition before starting your exercise program.

■ Assessing Your Level

After completing the Strength and Stretch Checks, you will know your levels for the exercises included in this chapter. If you scored in level 1, you probably have not exercised in a long time and your body is deconditioned. That's okay. We'll start out slowly, working to incorporate strength training twice each week into your Plan A and Plan B and get you ready to move on to levels 2 and 3. Here's some good news: because your body is unaccustomed to regular physical activity, you will see fast results—in about two to three weeks.

Scoring in level 2 indicates that you are in moderately good shape but probably don't exercise on a regular basis. You'll go at the workout harder and get into the habit of twice a week strength training.

Work Sheet 1: The Strength Check

The Strength Check should not be completed on the same day as the Heart Check from Chapter 8 (see page 209) because both tests may tire your legs, rendering the results of one of the checks inaccurate.

1. To perform the Strength Check, you will need: a sturdy wall; comfortable clothes; supportive sneakers; and a clock or watch with a second hand or a stopwatch. Warm up by walking briskly with your knees high for two to three minutes, followed by two minutes of gentle stretching.

2. Holding your timer (or where you can see the clock), stand with your back and shoulders leaning against the wall. Set your feet as wide apart as your shoulders. If you find it uncomfortable to place your back and shoulders against a bare wall, drape a thick towel over your back before continuing.

3. Looking straight ahead, walk your feet forward and let your butt slide down the wall, bending your knees until your thighs are parallel to the ground (or as low as you can if you can't get that far). Adjust your feet so that your knees are directly above your ankles, behind your tied shoelaces.

4. Breathe. And don't use your arms to help hold your position, just your legs. Keep your shoulders and upper back flat against the wall.

5. Check the time as soon as you get into position. Hold it for as long as you can and note the time.

Starting time: _____

Ending time: _____

Time held (in seconds): _____

Results:

Couldn't get to parallel	Level 1
Less than a minute	Level 1
60 to 90 seconds	Level 2
More than 90 seconds	Level 3

Strength Check Level: _____

Work Sheet 2: The Stretch Check

There is a small risk of muscular strain if you lean forward too quickly or forcefully. Before you begin this test, warm up by walking briskly for two to three minutes, followed by gentle stretching of the lower back. Perform the Stretch Check very slowly and cautiously. (See the egg stretch on page 247.)

1. To perform the Stretch Check, you will need: comfortable clothes; floor space.
2. Sit on the floor with your legs spread in a V so that your heels are about twelve inches apart. Sit up tall, through the top of your head, with your back straight and your head up, shoulders back.
3. If you can't sit in this position without bending your knees or if you feel pain in your lower back or along the backs of your legs, stop. Mark yourself down as level 1.
4. If you're doing okay at this point, take a few deep breaths. Keeping your back straight, put your arms out in front of you with your thumbs touching and your fingers extending forward. Inhale.
5. Without curving your back, exhale and reach your fingertips as far forward as you can without pain.
6. Hold the stretch for about ten seconds and make a mental note of how far you went along your legs with your fingertips.

Position reached: _____

Results:

Between waist and knee	Level 1
Below knee to midshin	Level 2
Lower shin to toes or beyond	Level 3

Stretch Check Level: _____

Again because your body is unaccustomed to *regular* activity, you should see your progress about a month after you get started.

If you scored in level 3, you're in good shape and probably exercising regularly. To continue receiving the benefits of strength training, you need to carefully examine your workout intensity to make sure you remain challenged and keep improving. If your body is already conditioned to strength training, with increased vigor and intensity in your workout you can expect to see a difference in six to eight weeks.

Whatever your current level, you need to commit to continually refining your Plan A fitness routine. It's vital for longevity but especially for stress reduction. Many of my patients initially found exercising regularly awkward and difficult. Most, however, have grown to love it with time, and while some say they still find it tedious, they notice the difference in their bodies and minds if they miss a workout. For instance, my Stress Undereaters feel anxious and agitated without their regular workouts. My Stress Overeaters feel a significant decline in energy and an increase in depression and hopelessness when they do not exercise regularly.

The bottom line is that regular physical activity is the best natural antidepressant available to women, particularly at the time of perimenopause. All of my patients have learned to appreciate how good it actually feels. As with Naomi, they feel stronger, more energetic, more capable, and happier. Moreover, as women become physically stronger, I have noticed that they have become mentally more stress resilient.

When I first met Linda, she was forty-nine years old. At five feet, four inches tall, she weighed 230 pounds. Linda sought me out for the usual reason: I was the doctor of last resort. During our first visit, I told Linda that she would be walking on her treadmill five or six times a week and strength training twice a week. She looked at me and said, "Look, I'm going to be honest with you. I hate to exercise, but I'm going to do it because I trust you." And with a smile on her face, Linda left my office to begin her journey.

Eleven later months later, at Christmastime, Linda was 45 pounds lighter and quite fit. When she came to see me for her appointment, Linda said, "I have a Christmas present for you." As I looked around for a box with a red ribbon on it, Linda said, "No, Dr. Peeke. My present for you is something I'm going to say. . . . As a result of working with you, I now hate exercise less!" This was one of the best presents I have ever gotten—when a sedentary, sad, unfit woman blossoms into an energetic and fit human being.

■ The KISS (Keep It Sublimely Simple) Home Workout Plan

Because you have committed to exercise, you need a few things to get started.

1. **Begin by purchasing three sets of dumbbells, in 3-, 5-, and 8-pound increments. If you are at level 3 and want to pick up a pair of 10-pound weights, go for it! You will also need one set each of 3- and 5-pound ankle weights.**
2. **Find a place within your home where you can work out; you will need enough room to lie down on the floor. Also make sure you have a towel and sturdy chair.**
3. **Dress in comfortable clothes and a pair of sneakers.**

The strength-training routine that follows should be viewed as a primer for the average over-forty woman who is just beginning to add regular physical activity to her daily life. This routine is not meant for people who are already advanced in weight training, although most of the exercises shown are the core building blocks of anyone's strength-training routine. Since this is an introductory weight-training routine, it may become fairly easy for you in a matter of months. At that time, you will need to regroup and increase the intensity of your strength workouts so you remain challenged. This can be accomplished in a number of ways. You can

- **Increase the amount of weight you are using**
- **Increase the number of repetitions, or reps (one complete movement of an exercise)**
- **Increase the number of sets (fixed number of repetitions; e.g., fifteen reps may comprise one set)**

If you feel unsure of yourself at any point, you may decide you want to schedule a session or two with a personal trainer or join a gym for further guidance.

■ Fitness over Forty Rules

First, avoid dehydration by drinking plenty of fluids during exercise. Hot or humid conditions make it difficult for the body to shed the excess heat generated by exercise, and that can result in a rapid increase in body temperature. Time your workouts for the cooler times of day. Increase your fluid intake and go at a slower pace when it is warm.

Progress slowly over time to allow your body the chance to rest, rebuild, and strengthen. Never try to lift a weight that you do not feel comfortable with. Begin at your predetermined level, keep consistent, and your goal of increased muscles and strength is well within your reach.

■ Flexibility Training

Flexibility training, as I explained in Chapter 8, is the third component of a well-balanced exercise plan. Please, do not skip the stretching! I found out the hard way just how necessary it is. In 1998, spurred on by the success of Oprah and some of my very own patients, I decided to run the Marine Corps marathon. For seven months, I trained hard for the actual run but did not stretch enough and I felt that neglect in my tightening hamstrings during every step of the last five miles of the race. My thighs were painfully tight, limiting my movement, and made those last miles an unnecessary trial. In preparation for running the New York marathon, I have made flexibility my new middle name. Many of us skip stretching because we feel we don't have time. But it is vital to health and self-sufficiency as you age. Tight muscles are very limiting as they don't extend as far as you might want to reach.

The main reason we become less flexible as we get older is a result of certain changes that take place in our connective tissues. As we age, our bodies gradually dehydrate to some extent. This absolutely does not mean that you should give up trying to achieve flexibility if you scored a level 1 on the Stretch Check and you feel you have always been inflexible. This just means that you will have to work harder, *and more carefully,* over a longer period of time as you gradually increase your flexibility and, therefore, your mobility. Remember, increases in the ability of your muscles and connective tissues to elongate (stretch) can be achieved at any age. Stretching stimulates the production and/or the retention of vital joint lubricants (like synovial fluid) between our connective tissues and helps prevent the formation of nasty adhesions that will slow you down.

Stretching will become even more important to you as you begin your exercise program. Without stretching, you lose some of your flexibility as you increase your muscle mass. And tight muscles are thought to be more prone to injury than stretched ones. That has certainly been my experience. If I work out a lot and do not spend enough time stretching, I end up with funny pains—in my knees, my lower back, and other spots. But if I do a little extra stretching whenever I work out, I feel really mobile. And that's one of your goals: to keep moving.

Strength training and flexibility training go hand in hand. It is a common misconception that there must always be a trade-off between flexibility and strength. The reality is that flexibility training and strength training actually enhance one another.

■ When to Stretch

One of the best times to stretch is right after your strength-training exercises. Stretching your fatigued muscles immediately following the exercise that caused the fatigue helps increase your flexibility, enhances the promotion of muscle growth, and will help decrease your level of postexercise soreness. Here's why: After you have lifted weights to fatigue your muscles, your muscles remain somewhat shortened, even though you are done with the movement and have stopped the exercise. This muscle shortening is due to the repetitive movement of your muscles against resistance. Body builders call this getting "pumped." Your "pumped" muscle is also full of lactic acid and other chemical by-products from exercising. If your muscle is not stretched afterward, it will stay slightly shortened, in this decreased range of motion. Think of it like your muscle is forgetting how to make itself as long as it could be. Static (nonbouncing) stretching of the muscle helps it to become looser and to gently ease it back into its full range of motion.

To maximize the time spent on your strength-training workout, I have integrated stretching into the exercise program. This will also help you to feel how stretching is the perfect complement to flexing your muscles. Get used to stretching your body so it feels nice and loose and ready to move! When done properly, stretching can do more than just increase flexibility. Some great benefits of stretching include

- **Enhanced physical fitness and ability to learn and perform skilled movements**
- **Increased mental and physical relaxation**
- **Enhanced development of body awareness**
- **Reduced risk of injury to joints, muscles, and tendons**
- **Reduced muscular soreness and tension**
- **Increased suppleness due to stimulation of the production of chemicals that lubricate connective tissues**

Some of the most common mistakes made when stretching are improper warm-up, inadequate rest between workouts, overstretching, performing the wrong exercises, and performing exercises in the wrong (or suboptimal) order.

■ The Importance of Warming Up

Stretching is not warming up! It is, however, a very important part of warming up. Warming up is quite literally the process of raising your core body temperature. It is very important that you perform a general warm-up before you stretch. Do not stretch before your muscles are warm. Warming up can do more than just loosen stiff muscles; when done properly, it can actually improve performance. On the other hand, an improper warm-up, or no warm-up, can greatly increase your risk of injury from engaging in physical activities.

To warm up, you should engage in at least five minutes of aerobic activity, such as brisk walking or any other activity that will cause a similar increase in your cardiovascular output (i.e., get your blood pumping). Increased blood flow in the muscles improves muscle performance and flexibility and reduces the likelihood of injury. Follow this activity with gentle stretching to complete your warm-up.

It is very important not to try to increase flexibility too quickly by forcing yourself. Stretch no farther than the muscles will go without pain. One of the easiest ways to overstretch is to stretch "cold" (without any warm-up). Even when you stretch properly, you may feel some discomfort. One way to think of it is if, while you are stretching, you feel like saying "ouch!," then you should ease up immediately and stop the stretch. Stretching correctly means that you definitely feel the tension in your muscle, and perhaps even light, gradual pins and needles; but if it becomes sudden, sharp, or uncomfortable, then you are overdoing it.

With enough stretching, flexibility can be developed no matter what level you started at. I do not mean to imply, however, that flexibility can be developed at the same rate by everyone. If you scored a level 1, it will take you a little longer to develop the desired level of flexibility. This means you must be more patient with yourself if you scored a level 1 and not push the stretch to the point of pain.

■ Don't Forget to Breathe!

I have included breathing instructions for each exercise that follows, as many people forget to breathe when they are doing strength workouts. It's also tempting to hold your breath and let the extra pressure help the lift, but that can raise your blood pressure dangerously and damage your eardrums. Plus, breathing deeply while you push weights around will definitely reduce stress. It's a great way to literally "blow off" steam.

Don't get nervous about breathing incorrectly—any breathing is good. But the particular inhales and exhales can help with pacing. And because you tend to tighten your abdominal muscles a bit when you exhale, if done during the hard part of the move, it can help keep your form precise. Give it a try. You will need to allow yourself time to practice this breathing but after a month or two you will find that it has become second nature during your strength-training routine.

■ The Workout

Here are the strength-training exercises I recommend for the average over-forty woman. For each exercise I have noted which muscle groups are being worked. Refer to the diagram of muscle groups in Appendix D so you can picture each muscle working as you complete a movement. It is wonderful to feel your muscles getting stronger and stronger as the weeks go by.

After the exercises, I have included a table based on the Strength Check that explains the appropriate number of repetitions for each exercise at each level. For some exercises, you will be doing multiple sets, or groups of repetitions. Each set should be separated by a fifteen- to thirty-second break to give your muscles a brief chance to rest. This is the perfect time to complete the stretches associated with each exercise.

It is important to complete these exercises in the order shown, in- cluding the stretches. Your workout begins with the large muscle groups of the body, the legs, chest, and back. Then you progress to the middle-sized muscle groups of the shoulders and abdomen. Your workout finishes with the smaller muscles in your arms—your biceps and triceps. If you start in the wrong place or skip around, the rou- tine will not be as effective for you, and you may not see the results you want. I also recommend doing these in a place where you can check your form in a mirror. If that is not possible for every work- out, check each move in a mirror every two weeks or ask someone to check your form and compare it with the photos that accompany the exercises.

It is also important to warm up your muscles before each strength-training workout. You can do this by taking a five-minute walk around the block or on a treadmill. You may want to incorpo- rate weight training after you do your cardiovascular routine so you are nice and warmed up before you start. If you choose this option, take care that you are not too tired to pay attention to your form dur- ing the strength training. After you are thoroughly warmed up, here's what to do.

■ Bum-Busting Squats and Standing Quadriceps Stretch

This exercise works your gluteus maximus (*butt*) muscles as well as your quadriceps femoris (*front of your upper thigh*) and biceps femoris (back of your upper thigh, also called hamstrings).

1. **Stand with your feet shoulder width apart and arms extended in front of you at shoulder height.**

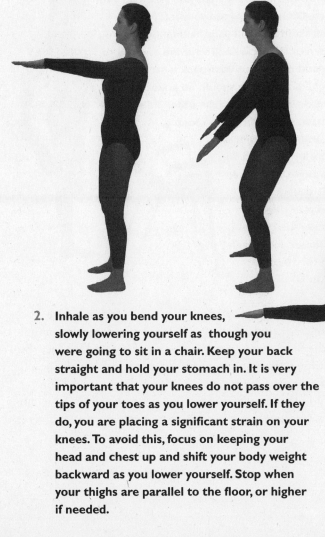

2. **Inhale as you bend your knees, slowly lowering yourself as though you were going to sit in a chair. Keep your back straight and hold your stomach in. It is very important that your knees do not pass over the tips of your toes as you lower yourself. If they do, you are placing a significant strain on your knees. To avoid this, focus on keeping your head and chest up and shift your body weight backward as you lower yourself. Stop when your thighs are parallel to the floor, or higher if needed.**

3. **When your thighs are parallel to the floor, exhale while you raise yourself back to the starting position. Try to imagine pressing up through the heels, not the toes, and squeeze your butt like a fist as you press up through the heels and exhale. If getting your thighs parallel to the floor is too hard, do a three-quarter squat—don't lower your butt down as far. If you are concerned about falling, do your squats in front of a soft sturdy chair or couch that can catch you.**

4. **Stretch break! At the conclusion of your set, hold on to the back of a chair and stand on your right leg. Grab the ankle of your left leg with your left hand and pull your heel up behind you toward your buttock. Keep your knees close together and make sure your back is straight, not arched. Your knee should be pointing straight down. Repeat on the other side. If you have a knee limitation, loop a towel around your foot and keep the leg bent at a 90-degree angle. You should feel this stretch in the front of your thigh, not your knee—be gentle with yourself. Hold each stretch for 10 to 30 seconds.**

■ Dumbbell Press and Chest Stretch

This exercise works the pectoralis major (*chest*), the *triceps* (the back
of your arms), and the *deltoids* (shoulders).

1. Lie on your back on the floor or on an exercise bench with your
    knees raised and feet flat on the floor. Hold the dumbbell on
    either side of your chest, elbows extended, palms facing forward.
    Your hands should be placed knuckles up, midchest. Imagine
    that you are holding a bar or broomstick in your hands.

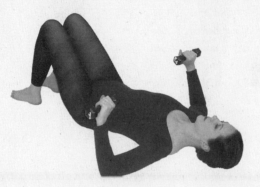

2. Take a deep breath.
3. As you exhale, press the weights up at a slight angle until your
    arms are almost straight. Imagine that you are making a trian-
    gle over your chest as you press upward. Hold a moment, then
    lower the weights to chest level.

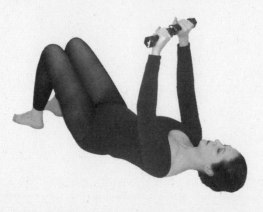

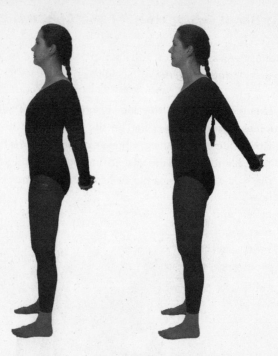

4. **At the conclusion of each set, stop and stretch out your chest and arms by sitting or standing with your hands clasped behind your back, fingers interlaced, palms turned inward. With your shoulder blades squeezed together and your shoulders pressing down toward the floor, lift your arms up behind you, leaning slightly forward, as you press your chest gently forward until you feel a stretch in your upper chest and shoulders. Hold the stretch for 10 to 30 seconds.**

■ Dumbbell Row and Straight Arm Shoulder Stretch

This exercise works your latissimus dorsi, teres major, and trapezius muscles (*back*) and also uses your deltoids (*shoulders*) and *biceps* (the front of the top of your arms). The dumbbell row is the complementary exercise to the dumbbell press. It will help to tighten up that often flabby area around your bra straps in the back.

1. Place your right knee and hand on a stool, bench, or couch and bend forward so that your back is flat and almost parallel to the floor. Hold your stomach in. It is very, very important that your back is flat; have a friend or exercise buddy check your form if you can or do this where you can see yourself in a mirror by turning your head slightly to the side.

2. Grasp the dumbbell in your left hand and let your left arm hang toward the floor. Your chest should almost be parallel to the floor. Don't let your arm dangle down too low or you will find that your shoulder dips down toward the floor.

3. Inhale as you slowly bend your arm, lifting the weight to hip level and keeping it close to your body. Your elbow should be pointing straight up toward the ceiling.

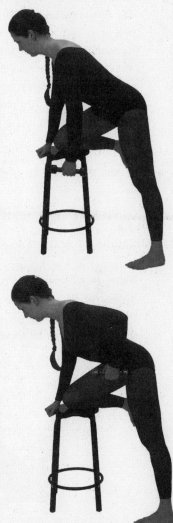

4. Hold for a moment, then exhale as you slowly lower the weight.
5. Repeat using the right arm.
6. At the conclusion of each set, it's stretch time! Place your left arm across your chest, keeping your arm straight and your shoulders down. Bring your right arm up from underneath; place it just above the elbow of the left arm and actively but gently pull your left arm toward your body. Repeat for the other side. You should feel this stretch across the top of your shoulder and upper arm. Hold this stretch for 10 to 30 seconds.

■ Bent-Knee Push-up

This exercise works your pectoralis major (*chest*) and *triceps* (the back of your upper arms), but should be avoided if you have carpal tunnel syndrome or other wrist problems.

1. Begin on all fours with your hands directly beneath your shoulders. This exercise is best done on a towel or a comfortable rug.
2. Raise your feet, ankles crossed.

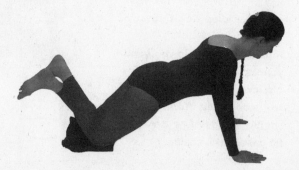

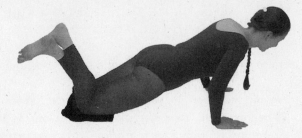

3. Inhale as you slowly lower your chest until it is a few inches off the floor. It is very, very important to hold your stomach in and keep your back flat. Perhaps a friend or exercise buddy could check out your back or you could find a place where you could look sideways into a mirror to check it yourself.

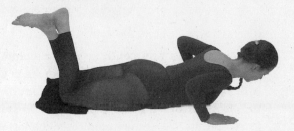

4. Exhale as you push yourself back up until your arms are almost straight.
5. At the conclusion of your set, sit or stand up and do the *chest stretch* (see page 242) as shown above.

■ Toxic Waist-Busting Curl-up and Egg Stretch (Lower Back Knee Hug)

This exercise works your rectus abdominis (*stomach*) muscles.

1. **Lie on the floor on your back with your knees bent at a 90-degree angle. Your feet should be flat on the floor, about twelve inches from your buttocks. Cross your arms over your chest.**

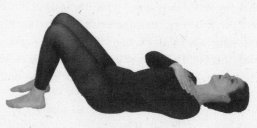

2. **Inhale as you slowly contract your abdominal muscles and raise your shoulder blades off the floor. Keep your head in line with your body. Try not to tense your neck or press your chin to your chest. Be very careful not to put pressure on your neck as you lift up. We women tend to hold a lot of tension in our necks. (Hint: Keeping your eyes on a spot high on the wall may help you maintain the right position. You can also imagine having a grapefruit under your chin.) You should feel the effort in your stomach area, not in your neck or lower back.**

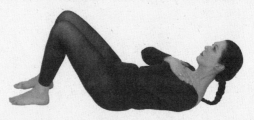

3. **Briefly hold the up position, then exhale as you slowly lower yourself back down to the floor.**
4. **If these do not feel good to you, do roll-downs instead. Start in the same position as the curl-up with a pillow under your head. Sit up, keeping your knees bent and feet flat on the floor in**

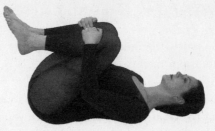

front of you. Reach your arms out in front of you. Firm your abdominal muscles with the one breath as done above. Then, on
the next exhale, roll your back down, then your shoulders and
finally your head onto the pillow.

5. At the completion of each set of abdominals, do the *egg stretch*.
Lie on your back with your knees bent and your feet flat on the
floor. Keeping your knees bent, tuck them into your chest and
reach around both legs and gently pull your thighs into your
chest, lifting your feet off the floor. Your legs should feel relaxed
throughout the entire move. You should feel this stretch in
your lower back and buttocks. I refer to this as the *egg stretch* because you will somewhat resemble an egg when doing this
stretch. Hold this position for 10 to 30 seconds.

■ Inner Thigh Leg Lifts and Groin Stretch

This exercise works the adductor group (*inner thighs*). The use of ankle weights is optional.

1. **Lie on your right side and rest your head on your right arm so as not to strain your neck. Straighten your right leg and cross your left leg in front of your right thigh so that your left foot is flat on the floor. Or if it feels more comfortable to you, rest your left leg gently on the floor as shown.**

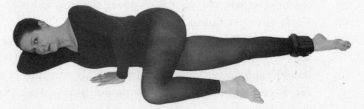

2. **Lift your left leg as high as you can, contracting (squeezing) the inner thigh, keeping your heel higher than your toes. Try not to feel a strain anywhere but in your inner thigh. Don't tense other parts of your body, particularly your neck.**

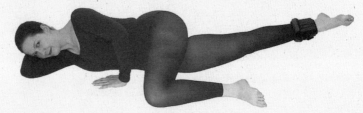

3. **Perform the appropriate number of repetitions (see How Many Do I Do?, page 255) and roll over and repeat with the right leg.**
4. **Take a stretch break after each set, performing the *groin stretch*. Sit up with the soles of your feet together; lean forward, keeping a normal lumbar curve in your back by sitting up tall. Pull your feet comfortably toward your body. Allow your knees to go toward the floor to stretch the inner thighs of both legs. If you are at level 2 or 3 for stretching, you may perform this stretch while you are lying on your back by gently pulling your feet in toward your groin by grasping your ankles.**

■ Side-Lying Leg Raises and Hamstring Stretches

This exercise works the gluteus maximus (*butt*) muscle, the iliopsoas, the tensor fasciae latae, and the abductor longus (*hips* and *outer thighs*). Use of ankle weights is optional.

1. Lie on your side and rest your head on your right arm so as not to strain your neck. Extend your legs in a straight line.
2. Bend your bottom leg at a 90-degree angle to give your body stability.

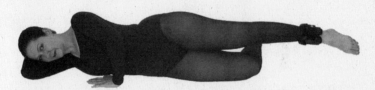

3. Lift your top leg to about hip height, keeping your entire leg taut and solid as you lift. Keep your back straight. Try not to feel a strain anywhere but in your outer thigh. Don't tense other parts of your body, particularly your neck.

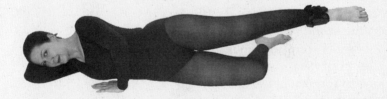

4. Lower your leg, but do not rest it until you have finished all of the repetitions. Do not rock your pelvis forward and backward as you lift and lower. Keep your abs tight.
5. Perform your set and then roll over and repeat with the other leg.
6. Take a stretch break after each set, using one of the hamstring stretches below.

■ Seated Hamstring Stretch

Sit with your legs straight in front of you, feet relaxed (do not flex or point them). Bend one leg so that the bottom of the foot touches the inner thigh of the straight leg. With a straight back and open chest, bring your forehead toward the shin of the straight leg. Reach for your foot with both hands. Hold each stretch for 10 to 30 seconds. Repeat for the other leg. If you cannot reach your foot, place a towel around the foot of the straight leg and hold on to the ends of the towel with both hands. You should feel this stretch in the back of your thigh. Again, hold each stretch for 10 to 30 seconds.

■ Lying Hamstring Stretch

Lie on your back with your knees bent and your feet flat on the floor. Extend one leg straight up toward the ceiling. Grasp that leg with both hands at the thigh or calf and slowly pull it toward your face until you feel a slight tension. Make sure you keep your head relaxed, with your chin tucked in slightly. The important thing is not how close your leg comes to your chest but that the leg stays straight and you feel tension. If you have difficulty reaching your leg, loop a towel around your foot for help. You should feel this stretch in the back of your thigh. Hold this stretch for 10 to 30 seconds. Repeat for the other leg.

■ Elvis-Pelvis Tilts

This exercise works your gluteus maximus (*butt*) muscles and your biceps femoris (the back of your upper thigh, also known as *hamstrings*).

1. **Lie on your back with your arms relaxed at your sides, knees bent, feet about shoulder width apart and heels on the floor.**

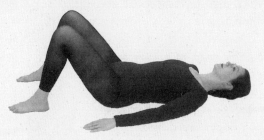

2. **With your shoulders back, squeeze your buttocks, raising your pelvis off the floor but keeping your upper back on the floor. Hold for 1 second, then lower.**

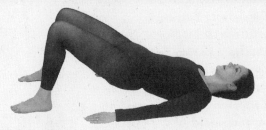

3. **Do the *egg stretch* (see page 247).**

■ Bench/Chair Dip

This exercise works both your deltoids (*shoulders*) and *triceps* (the back of the upper arms). It is very effective in treating a flabby underarm area. Be careful if you have any wrist limitations or shoulder problems. If you have any orthopedic limitations or if this exercise does not feel comfortable to you, skip it and go on to the *triceps extension* described below. Make certain that the bench or chair you use is **very sturdy** so that it doesn't tip over, potentially injuring you.

1. Sit on the edge of a very sturdy chair or bench, or even the bottom step of the staircase at home.

2. Grasping the seat with your fingertips pointing forward, inhale as you slowly lower your body toward the floor until your elbows are bent at right angles. It is extremely important to keep your butt close in to the chair. If you are too far away, you will place a strain on your shoulder joints. Don't lock your elbows, even at the top part of the movement.

3. Keeping your feet flat on the floor, exhale as you use the backs of your arms to push yourself back up to the starting position.

4. After each set, use the *straight arm shoulder stretch* (see page 243).

■ Triceps Extension and Triceps Stretch

This exercise works the back of your upper arm (*triceps*).

1. Hold dumbbell in your left hand, palm facing in.
2. Bend over until your upper body is almost parallel to the floor.
3. Place your right hand on your right knee.

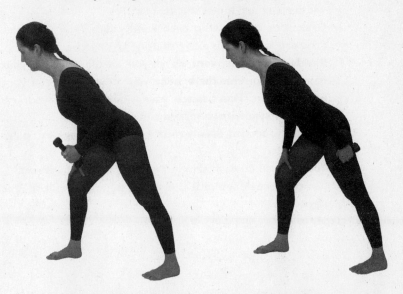

4. Press the dumbbell backward in a semicircular motion as you exhale, keeping your left elbow in the same position by your side.
5. Hold the dumbbell momentarily in that position.
6. As you inhale, slowly lower the dumbbell back to the starting position.
7. Following each set, stretch out your triceps by placing one hand behind your head between your shoulder blades. Leaving your arm in this position, very gently press your elbow toward your head using your other hand.
8. Repeat the strength training exercise and stretch with your other arm.

■ Double Biceps Curl

This exercise works the front of your upper arms (*biceps*), which are often the first area to show you your hard work. Your bicep is the muscle that pops out when you make a "Popeye muscle." Soon you will be showing your muscle all over town.

1. Stand with your arms at your sides, feet about a shoulder width apart and knees slightly bent.
2. Grasp one dumbbell in each hand, palms facing forward. (You can also do this exercise using an exercise band.)
3. Slowly bend your arms up as you exhale, bringing your hands to your shoulders. Keep your elbows still and your back straight. Don't brace your elbows against your rib cage. Keep your wrists locked and solid.
4. Hold for I second. Slowly return to the starting position as you inhale.
5. You can also do each arm individually, alternating them.
6. Conclude each set with the *straight arm shoulder stretch* (see page 243).

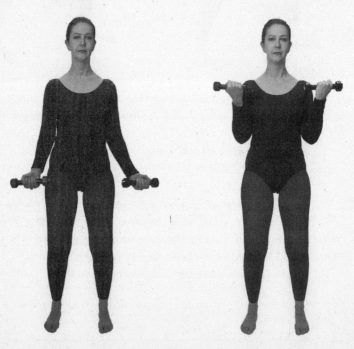

Table 9-1. **How Many Do I Do?: Strength Training**

Exercise	Level	Sets/ Repetitions	Suggested Weight*	Stretch (for each level, to follow each set)
Bum-busting squats	1	1 set/8 reps	—	Standing quadriceps stretch
	2	2 sets/10 reps each	—	
	3	3 sets/15–25 reps each	—	
Level 3: increase number of reps until you hit 25 per set				
Dumbbell press	1	1st set/10 reps	3 lbs.	Chest stretch
		2nd set/8 reps	5 lbs.	
	2	1st set/15 reps	5 lbs.	
		2nd set/10 reps	8 lbs.	
	3	1st set/15 reps	8 lbs.	
		2nd set/10 reps	10 lbs.	
Dumbbell row	1	1st set: 15 reps	3 lbs.	Straight arm shoulder stretch
		2nd set/10 reps	5 lbs.	
	2	1st set/15 reps	5 lbs.	
		2nd set/10 reps	8 lbs.	
	3	1st set/15 reps	8 lbs.	
		2nd set/10 reps	10 lbs.	
Do the suggested number of reps for each arm to comprise one set				
Bent-knee push-up	1	1 set/3–4 reps	—	Chest stretch
	2	1 set/10 reps	—	
	3	1st set/15 reps	—	
		2nd set/10 reps	—	
When looking for something more challenging, add 5 push-ups to your current amount before progressing to the next level				
Toxic Waist-busting curl-ups	1	1 set/25 reps	—	Egg stretch
	2	1st set/25	—	
		2nd set/25	—	
	3	1st set/25	—	
		2nd set/25	—	
		3rd set/25	—	

Exercise	Level	Sets/ Repetitions	Suggested Weight*	Stretch (for each level, to follow each set)
Inner thigh leg lifts	1	1 set/25	—	Groin stretch
	2	2 sets/25 reps	3 lbs. (ankle)	
	3	2 sets/25 reps	5 lbs. (ankle)	

All levels: for each exercise, perform 1 set for each leg

Level 2: before progressing to the next level, do first set with 5-lb. ankle weight, 2nd set with 3-lb. ankle weight

Level 3: when ready for a more challenging workout, a heavier ankle weight may be used

Exercise	Level	Sets/ Repetitions	Suggested Weight*	Stretch (for each level, to follow each set)
Side-lying leg raises	1	1 set/25 reps	—	Seated hamstring stretch or lying hamstring stretch
	2	2 sets/25 reps	3 lbs. (ankle)	
	3	2 sets/25 reps	5 lbs. (ankle)	

All levels: for each exercise, perform 1 set for each leg

Level 2: before progressing to the next level, do first set with 5-lb. ankle weight, 2nd set with 3-lb. ankle weight

Level 3: when ready for a more challenging workout, a heavier ankle weight can be used for the 1st set

Exercise	Level	Sets/ Repetitions	Suggested Weight*	Stretch (for each level, to follow each set)
Elvis-pelvis tilts	1	1 set/25 reps	—	Egg stretch
	2	2 sets/25 reps	—	
	3	3 sets/25 reps	—	
Bench/chair dip	1	1 set/4–5 reps	—	Straight arm shoulder stretch
	2	1 set/10 reps	—	
	3	1st set/10 reps	—	
		2nd set/10 reps		

Do not progress to more than 3 sets of 10 of this exercise

Exercise	Level	Sets/ Repetitions	Suggested Weight*	Stretch (for each level, to follow each set)
Triceps extension	1	1st set/15 reps	3 lbs.	Triceps stretch
		2nd set/10 reps	5 lbs.	
	2	1st set/15 reps	5 lbs.	
		2nd set/10 reps	8 lbs.	

Exercise	Level	Sets/ Repetitions	Suggested Weight*	Stretch (for each level, to follow each set)
Triceps extension	3	1st set/15 reps	8 lbs.	
(cont'd)		2nd set/10 reps	10 lbs.	

Perform 2 sets of this exercise for each arm; if the 2nd set seems too difficult, work up to it by repeating set 1 instead

Exercise	Level	Sets/ Repetitions	Suggested Weight*	Stretch (for each level, to follow each set)
Double bicep curls	1	1st set/15 reps	3 lbs.	Straight arm
		2nd set/10 reps	5 lbs.	shoulder stretch
	2	1st set/15 reps	5 lbs.	
		2nd set/10 reps	8 lbs.	
	3	1st set/15 reps	8 lbs.	
		2nd set/10 reps	10 lbs.	

All levels; if the 2nd set seems too difficult, work up to it by repeating set 1 instead

Level 3: you may do these one arm at a time if it feels too difficult for your last set

*Suggested weight: The weights listed here are suggestions only. To start out, use as much weight as feels comfortable for the first set of reps. The last rep of any exercise should feel fairly hard to perform. Pay very close attention to your form. Do not sacrifice correct form by trying to lift a weight that is too heavy for you. Use your first few workout sessions as testing sessions to see how much weight feels comfortable for you. Once you are able to complete all the sets of an exercise with the suggested weight and it feels almost easy, you are ready to advance to the next level for that specific exercise.

Table 9-2. **More About Stretching**

This table provides you with minimum recommendations to improve your flexibility. The stretches listed below should be completed following each set of the related exercise. If you scored at level 1 on the Stretch Check, even if you scored at level 2 or 3 on the Heart Check or the Strength Check, you will be doing a few more stretches than the other levels. All levels: remember to warm up thoroughly with at least 5 minutes of rhythmic aerobic activity before stretching—stretching is not warming up. If you want to do additional stretching, that is fabulous!

Exercise	Level 1 (Hold all stretches for at least 20 seconds)	Level 2	Level 3
Bum-busting squats	Standing quadriceps stretch: repeat the sequence (right, left, right, left)	Standing quadriceps stretch: hold for at least 20 seconds on each side	Standing quadriceps stretch
Dumbbell press	Chest stretch followed by straight arm shoulder stretch: repeat this sequence	Chest stretch followed by straight arm shoulder stretch	Chest stretch
Dumbbell row	Straight arm shoulder stretch followed by chest stretch: repeat this sequence	Straight arm shoulder stretch followed by chest stretch	Straight arm shoulder stretch
Bent-knee push-up	Chest stretch followed by shoulder moves* and then ballerina stretch*	Chest stretch followed by shoulder moves*	Chest stretch
Toxic Waist-busting	Egg stretch followed by	Egg stretch followed by	Egg stretch –

curl-ups	crossed ankle stretch:* repeat this sequence	crossed ankle stretch*	
Inner thigh leg lifts	Groin stretch: repeat	Groin stretch	Groin stretch
Side-lying leg raises	Hamstring stretch† followed by crossed ankle stretch:* repeat this sequence	Hamstring stretch† followed by crossed ankle stretch*	Hamstring stretch*
Elvis-pelvis tilts	Egg stretch followed by crossed ankle stretch*: repeat this sequence	Egg stretch followed by crossed ankle stretch*: repeat this sequence	Egg stretch
Bench/chair dip	Straight arm shoulder stretch followed by shoulder moves* and then ballerina stretch*: repeat this sequence	Straight arm shoulder stretch followed by shoulder moves* and then ballerina stretch*: repeat this sequence	Straight arm shoulder stretch followed by ballerina stretch*
Triceps extension	Triceps stretch followed by straight arm shoulder stretch: repeat this sequence	Triceps stretch	Triceps stretch
Double bicep curls	Straight arm shoulder stretch followed by chest stretch and then shoulder moves*: repeat this sequence	Straight arm shoulder stretch followed by chest stretch	Straight arm shoulder stretch

*These stretches are described later in Chapter 9.

†Choose either the seated hamstring stretch or the lying hamstring stretch.

I designed this workout so that you don't need a lot of equipment, but there are many wonderful exercises for gaining strength. The key is to have some kind of resistance for your muscles to work against. It can come from your body weight, dumbbells, ankle weights, exercise bands, barbells, weight machines, a medicine ball, or other sources. Not sure where to go for variety and direction?

■ A Note About Personal Training

Because strength workouts can be intense for the muscles being worked, it's easy to perform a move incorrectly. A personal trainer can monitor and correct your form as she or he knows what to look for. I would also recommend a session with a personal trainer when you get to the point where you want to vary your workouts or are looking for more of a challenge than level 3. If it's too expensive, see if you can get a group of people together to share the cost.

Finding a good personal trainer is like finding a good hairdresser or gynecologist—the best way to find one is by word of mouth. But buyer beware: because training is a combination of science and art, good trainers are hard to find. The safest trainers are those who have been certified by one of the top fitness organizations, such as the American College of Sports Medicine or the American Council on Exercise. Choose a trainer who is current with the latest news in exercise physiology, sports medicine, and nutrition. Your trainer should be dependable, creative, likable, and have experience working with the forty- to fifty-five-year-old woman. To find one, ask at a local health club, ask your friends, ask people at work, or call IDEA, the International Association of Fitness, at (619) 535-8979.

■ Stress-Reducing Stretches

As with your strength exercises, there are many other wonderful stretches in addition to those incorporated into your strength workout. As long as you keep your movements slow (no bouncing!) and keep breathing steadily, you can benefit from any stretch. Check out some of the great books and videos on stretching and go for it.

When it comes to stretching, Bob Anderson wrote the book on it—literally. His book, simply called *Stretching,* is excellent. There is also an accompanying video, *Stretching with Bob Anderson,* in which proper form is demonstrated. If your library or video store doesn't have it, you can get it for $20 from Collage, (800) 433-6769. Another excellent choice is Karen Voight's *Pure and Simple Stretch.* She demonstrates leg, butt, and arm moves at three levels.

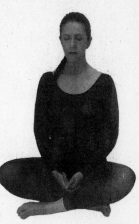

Yoga is also effective for building flexibility, balance, and strength. Several of the stretches in the workout above are based on yoga. For more information on yoga, check out a local class or try these videos: Kathy Smith's *New Yoga Basics* (flexibility poses, breathing, and relaxation); *P.M. Yoga for Beginners* (sunset views, relaxing poses); *Yoga Zone Introduction to Yoga* (deep breathing and basic moves); or *Lilias! Silver Yoga* (geared toward seniors).

Don't limit your stretching to a strength-training workout. It's a good idea to stretch your quadriceps and hamstrings before you go walking, for example. Stretching can also help relieve achy muscles. If your back ever aches, do the *egg stretch* (see page 247). You will also find stretching very relaxing. Some simple moves can be done to relieve tension while sitting at your desk or chasing the kids around the house.

Here are a few of my other favorite muscle relaxers. Include with these the stretch you performed in the Strength Check (see page 230) as it is great for the backs of your legs. The stretches below can be performed all at once, before or after your aerobic exercise, or incorporated into your strength-training workout.

Shoulder Moves (Loosens the shoulders.)

Do these sitting in a comfortable chair, preferably one with back support that comes up to your shoulder blades. First, slowly roll your shoulders front to back about 8 times and back to front another 8.

You shouldn't feel any pinching, but don't worry if your shoulders crackle as you roll them—that just means you need this! Next, scrunch your shoulders up toward your ears 8 times.

Crossed Arms (Loosens the upper back, rear of shoulders, and upper arms.)

Also do this one in a comfortable chair. Straighten your right arm and cross it in front of your chest. Grab your right wrist with your left hand, left elbow by your side. Rotate your right shoulder down (your right elbow will probably bend a little and your right hand will come up higher). Gently pull your right arm toward your left shoulder until you feel the stretch across the back of your right shoulder. Hold this position and breathe in and out for about 15 seconds. Switch sides and repeat. (If you have trouble sitting on a chair, do this stretch lying down.)

Ballerina Stretch (Loosens the chest, fronts of shoulders, and backs of upper arms.)

Sitting in a chair, clasp your hands together and lift your arms overhead. Sit up tall, hold your abdominal muscles tight, and push your hands as far back as you can without arching your back or tipping your head backward. Hold for 15 seconds and breathe. (If you have trouble sitting on a chair, do this stretch lying down, legs flat.)

Crossed Ankle (Loosens the backs of thighs, hips, and butt.)

Lie on the floor on your back, knees bent, feet flat on the ground. Lift your right leg and place the ankle on your left thigh, near the knee. Place your hands on either side of your left thigh and grasp it. Breathe out and gently pull your left foot off the floor, pulling the knee toward your shoulder as far as you comfortably can. Hold the stretch for 15 seconds, breathing. Slowly release. Switch sides and repeat. If you have trouble doing this stretch, go to a chair.

Cross your right thigh over your left. Exhale and reach for your toes. Hold the stretch and breathe.

Diamond Stretch (Loosens the hips and inner thighs.)

Lie on the floor with your knees bent, feet flat on the floor. Let your knees fall open to either side, the soles of your feet coming together. Straighten your back and reach for your feet. If you can reach them, hold on to your feet and try to press your knees out to either side without rounding your back. Hold and breathe for 15 seconds.

Calf Stretch (Loosens the calves and helps prevent shin splints.)

Stand with your legs a shoulder width apart. Take a large step forward with your left leg and then bend both knees slightly. Bend your torso forward, keeping your back straight, and place your hands on your left thigh for balance. Now slowly lower your right heel as far as you comfortably can. Hold for 15 seconds, breathing all the while. Switch sides and repeat. Adjust the intensity of the stretch by adjusting the size of your big step forward.

■ Stress Profile Exercise Prescriptions

Not every woman experiences life's stresses in the same way. By now you know this as well as your own unique stress profile. Stress Overeaters and Undereaters will most probably approach the beginning of their fitness journey differently. The exercise plans I prescribe should be customized and individualized to reflect your own stress profile needs. Clearly, all of the workouts are designed with the same goal in mind—to make you more Stress-Resilient!

First, let's look at a week in the life of a Stress-Resilient woman as she incorporates into her life her aerobic and strength training as well as stress-reducing habits.

Stress-Resilient

Day 1

> **Aerobic exercise: 45-minute walk outside or on a treadmill**
>
> **Midmorning stress reliever: 5-minute relaxation response exercise**
>
> **Extra physical activity for the day: took stairs instead of elevator (four flights)**
>
> **Midafternoon stretch break: stretched upper back and shoulders while at computer**
>
> **Evening stress reliever: 5-minute relaxation response exercise before bed**

Day 2

> **Aerobic exercise: 45-minute run or walk outside or on a treadmill**
>
> **Midmorning stress reliever: 5-minute walk around block outside of office**
>
> **Midafternoon stretch break: gently stretched legs and shoulders**
>
> **Extra physical activity for the day: took children to the park, ran with them instead of sitting**
>
> **Evening stress reliever: 10-minute bath with great smelling bubble bath**

Day 3

> **Aerobic exercise: 25-minute run or walk outside or on a treadmill**
>
> **Midmorning stress reliever: closed office doors, closed eyes, listened to music (5 minutes)**
>
> **Lunchtime exercise: 15-minute brisk walk near office**

Extra physical activity for the day: none
Strength training: completed entire strength-training routine
Evening stress reliever: completed extra stretches for 20 minutes

Day 4

Aerobic exercise: 45-minute run or walk outside or on a treadmill with a girlfriend
Midmorning stress reliever: elicited relaxation response (5 minutes)
Extra physical activity for the day: played a game with myself—vowed not to E-mail onsite colleagues; instead I walked to their offices
Midafternoon stress reliever: called a girlfriend and giggled (5 minutes)
Evening stress reliever: did 50 extra Toxic Waist-busting curl-ups (shown on page 246)

Day 5

Aerobic exercise: 25-minute brisk walk outdoors or on a treadmill
Midmorning stress reliever: elicited relaxation response through diaphragmatic breathing
Extra physical activity for the day: conscious stair climbing
Midafternoon stress reliever: 15-minute brisk walk around office with colleague
Evening stress reliever: strength-training routine (30 minutes)

Day 6

Aerobic exercise: 60-minute brisk walk outside with spouse or friend
Midmorning stress reliever: 5-minute relaxation response exercise

Lunchtime exercise: bike ride with the kids around the block
Extra physical activity for the day: tried a yoga class at the local
gym
Evening stress reliever: played with the dog (5 minutes)

Day 7

Aerobic exercise: took the kids hiking
Midmorning stress reliever: 5-minute relaxation response ex-
ercise
Lunchtime exercise: golf lesson
Extra physical activity for the day: none
Evening stress reliever: performed extra stretching routine for
30 minutes; taught spouse some stretches while watching
movies

Stress Overeaters

Stress Overeaters need more energy, or "activation," to cope with Toxic Stress. Therefore, the Stress Overeater's workout program includes a variety of energizing aerobic activities. I like to call these activities flight simulators because they represent the "flight" component of the "fight-or-flight" reaction to stress. Instead of running from a tiger, you are walking briskly on a treadmill. You need regular aerobic exercise to maintain higher levels of energy throughout the day.

In the parlance of the stress response, strength training is "fight simulation" of the "fight-or-flight" response since you will be using your muscles to lift, push, and pull to fight for your life. Here are two examples of how the "fight-or-flight" simulation might work:

Stress Overeater Flight Simulation:
Aerobic activity performed 5 to 6 times per week for 40 minutes, with 5 minutes of stretching on either end.

Stress Overeater Fight Simulation:
Strength-training activity two nonconsecutive days per week, 30 to 40 minutes, incorporating stretches after each exercise as shown above.

Even on rest days, Stress Overeaters must try to maintain a higher level of energy or activation. Take the kids on a hike through the woods. Pull out that dusty tennis racquet and go out with a girl-friend to hit balls. Go swimming. Go for a bike ride. Have some fun, even on days when you don't feel like vigorous physical activity. Simply get up and move. Make like a tourist in your own hometown and walk around and see what there is to see!

Stress Undereaters

Stress Undereaters tend to be more agitated and anxious when they wake up in the morning and often remain so throughout the day. Stress Undereaters need more calming activities to balance their nervous energy. Therefore, during aerobic physical activity, it is good to focus on becoming more mindful and aware of your breathing and body sensations to allow your mind to rest and relax with more calming thoughts. Here are two examples of how the "fight-or-flight" simulation might work for the Stress Undereater:

> Stress Undereater Flight Simulation:
> Aerobic activity performed 5 times per week for 40 minutes, with 5 minutes of stretching on either end.

> Stress Undereater Fight Simulation:
> Strength-training activity 2 times per week, 30 to 40 minutes each session, focusing on breathing, posture, and alignment. Work on clearing your mind during these sessions. Focus on breathing out, how the weight feels in your hands, how your muscles and body feel in motion. (I know, you are constantly in motion! But have you ever been mindful of the feeling you have as your body moves? It's delightful.)

■ Practicing the Fine Art of Regrouping

Exercise provides a beautiful opportunity to practice the art of regrouping, as you will constantly face obstacles that interfere with your exercise time. Think of these obstacles as opportunities to ex-

Muscle Recovery Plan

Some amount of soreness can be expected after your strength-training workouts, particularly as you start out or adjust your levels. Recall how muscles work. When you strength train, you do some small amount of damage to your muscle fibers. This encourages new muscle fibers to grow, causing your muscles to get bigger and stronger. The soreness you feel may be attributable to this damage.

You can, however, also overdo your workouts. If you have any sharp or persistent pains, especially in your joints, contact your doctor immediately.

But assuming the soreness you feel is the muscle rebuilding process, be proud! Your muscles are responding to your hard work. And there's a lot you can do to feel better until the pain goes away. Do any or all of the following:

- Drink a lot of water to help keep your body working in top condition. Water can help your body flush out the by-products of muscle damage.
- Get some sleep. This is prime body-healing time.
- Check with your doctor to see if you can take a painkiller such as Advil or Aleve as directed. These are effective for muscle pain.
- If one spot is very sore, ice it for the first forty-eight hours and use a hot-water bottle or heating pad on it after that. If your whole body is mildly achy (and you don't have any intensely painful spots), soak in a warm bath with Epsom salts. The warmth increases circulation, which helps in healing.
- If one spot is achy, try to keep it elevated. For example, sore thighs: put your legs up on a chair. This assists with blood flow and healing.
- Wear something snug. "Compression" aids healing because it helps blood flow. I'm not talking about those jeans that you need to jump up and down to get into. If your legs are sore, try snug-fitting leggings or pantyhose. If your arms are sore, try a long-sleeved leotard. The warmth of these clothes also helps.
- Get a massage. A massage by a nationally certified massage therapist will increase circulation in both your skin and muscles, encourage your muscle cells to release accumulated metabolic waste products into your bloodstream to be filtered out of your body, and relax you mentally as well as physically. You worked hard—pamper yourself!

pand your creativity; practice regrouping here and it will be easier to apply these skills to other areas of your life. If Plan A consists of getting to the gym on your way home from work at 5 P.M. but you don't get out of work until 7 P.M. and you are too exhausted to move, you need to go to Plan B. You can handle this.

One of my patients, Carrie, leads a lifestyle common to the over-forty woman. She has family, work, and community obligations to balance along with her self-care needs. Her current list includes two teenage children with activities she loves to attend and a husband with whom she wants to spend more time but their busy schedules often get in the way. Carrie has a demanding job as a writer and she faces unyielding deadlines, an overbearing, stress-inducing boss, and frequent travel obligations to conduct interviews. She also has friends and co-workers whom she likes to visit from time to time.

When she first came to see me at the age of forty-two, she was a Stress Overeater and facing frequent fatigue. In addition to understanding and incorporating the principles of the Nutrition Template into her daily life, Carrie also began exercising. At first she found it difficult to get up and get moving, but she loved the energy that her early-in-the-day exercise provided her with throughout the day. But remember Carrie's schedule, and you might guess that's not always possible. See on pages 270 and 271 how Carrie fits in her over-forty exercise during a typical week, shifting as necessary between Plan A and Plan B to balance her self-care and other commitments.

After having read Chapters 8 and 9, it should be apparent to anyone over the age of forty that physical activity is a nonnegotiable fact of life, not unlike brushing your teeth or taking a shower. This is especially true for women. The good news is that the expanding waistline and the accumulating body fat of the over-forty woman can definitely be controlled. Furthermore, it has to be controlled to save your life.

The solution is no longer a fad diet or an extreme exercise program. Neither of these can be sustained healthfully for life, and both create Toxic Stress, which will inevitably add more weight. The days of these crisis-oriented "wellness binges" have to stop in order to achieve the balanced mind and body you are seeking so desperately.

You now see that getting physical will

Monday
Plan A

6:20–7:15 A.M.	stretching/warm-up	5 minutes
	walks on treadmill	45 minutes (provides activation throughout the day)
	cool down	5 minutes

Tuesday
Plan B: boss called Monday night and Carrie must be available for 7:30 A.M. breakfast meeting

10:15–10:30 A.M.	walks around the block with co-worker	15 minutes (relieves stress from meeting)
12:55–1:00 P.M.	climbs stairs in her building between lunch and interview	5 minutes
5:30–5:40 P.M.	jogs to catch her bus	10 minutes
7:30–7:45 P.M.	takes her dog for a brief run	15 minutes (meets goal of 45 minutes of accrued exercise)

Wednesday
Plan A

| 6:30–7:15 A.M. | has session with personal trainer | completes one half of strength-training needs for week |
| 8:00–8:45 P.M. | walks around neighborhood with husband | 45 minutes |

Thursday
Plan B: travel

| 8:00–8:45 P.M. | uses stair climber and exercise bike in hotel gym | 45 minutes |
| 9:00–9:20 P.M. | performs additional stretching routine | 20 minutes (feels relaxed, mentally and physically) |

Friday
Day Off

Saturday

Plan B: attending daughter's tennis tournament in morning; visiting relatives in afternoon

8:00–8:15 A.M.	jogs with daughter while she warms up for match	15 minutes
5:30–5:40 P.M. 6:00–6:10 P.M.	walks to and from grocery store with son to buy ingredients for dinner	20 minutes
8:30–8:45 P.M.	stretching/warm-up walks on treadmill	5 minutes 10 minutes (meets goal of 45 minutes of accrued exercise)

Sunday

Plan B: church barbecue; gym is closed for annual cleaning

11:30–11:50 A.M.	walks around church grounds during break in set-up	20 minutes
4:30–5:00 P.M.	stretching/warm-up walks on treadmill	5 minutes 25 minutes (meets goal of 45 minutes of accrued exercise)
7:30–8:15 P.M.	home strength-training workout	completes strength-training needs for week

Keep those stress hormones in check
Eliminate Toxic Stress
Make you fit and firm
Prevent the accumulation of Toxic Weight
Add quality and longevity to your life

Years of dieting only served to foster a toxic mind-body dissociation. Moving your body begins a healing process that will keep your mind and body linked, working together harmoniously for life.

10 Putting It All Together

By now you realize that the three essential components of your wellness journey include:

- ✔ **Your mind: Stress-Resilient Regrouping**
- ✔ **Your eating: High-Quality/Low-Stress Foods**
- ✔ **Your body: Stress-Reducing Physical Activity**

From Part One of this book, you also are aware that you have a tendency to either overeat or undereat when typical daily stresses occur. You know your stress profile, and you know that the ultimate goal is the achievement of Stress-Resilient eating habits. To shed your after-forty fat and achieve your optimal level of wellness, you need to put it all together.

In the following stress prescriptions are recommendations regarding attitude (mind), nutrition (eating), and physical activity (body) for each stress profile. In addition, I have added some notes about specific herbal remedies that can be used to augment your program, soothe you, and keep your stress hormone levels as close to normal as possible.

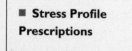
■ **Stress Profile Prescriptions**

The key is to aim for a lifestyle that supports Stress Resilience. We know that this is the Holy Grail of your quest to achieve the best level of wellness you can, and also shed your toxic mental and physical weight. You now have the tools to cope with the stresses that kept you from health and longevity. Fit, healthy, and happy, you can now open vistas of opportunities and enjoy your life's journey.

Box 10-1. **Rx for Stress-Resilient Women**

Goal	Maintaining a healthy level of balance in daily life.
	Objective: Practice stress-neutralizing behavior throughout the day.
Resilient attitude	Seek ways to practice and refine the process of re-grouping from daily stresses. Integrate stress into life; do not avoid it. See maintaining mental and physical vigor as essential. Living by the natural bio-rhythm of the stress hormones allows you to continue to plan and be prepared for the CortiZone.
Resilient eating	Avoid refined sugars. Maintain portion control. Prioritize High-Quality/Low-Stress foods that include fruits and vegetables as well as high-fiber starches (brown bread, whole wheat pasta, brown rice). Be mindful of the Carb Clock. Try to eliminate any starch after 5 P.M.
Physical activity	Move your body as an integral part of living; physical activity throughout the day will allow you to neutralize the stress response. Forty-five minutes of daily aerobic activity combined with strength training with weights twice per week should be your routine. Continue to challenge with new ways to achieve your daily physical activity. Turn off the day's stresses through mindful meditation and decrease obsession and worry.
Restorative herbs	Use herbs to naturally soothe and rebalance your stress system: vervain, skullcap, wild oat, black cohosh, ginseng, rosemary, ginger, lemon balm, and wood betony.

Box 10-2. **Rx for Stress Overeaters**

Goal	Maintaining a healthy level of energy and focus. *Objective:* Avoid stress overeating in the CortiZone.
Focused attitude	Realize that food is not an anesthetic; the pain of daily life is to be felt and integrated into life. Learn to regroup and move between Plan A (routine) and Plan B (routine under stress). Realize that reward comes, not from overconsumption of food but from living a rich and fulfilling life. Meditation through the Relaxation Response is helpful to lessen the acute pain of daily stresses.
Focused eating	Plan your meals well ahead of time to avoid mindless quick hunger fixes.
	Avoid refined sugars.
	Avoid family-sized food bags, cartons, and boxes.
	Turn your world into a single-serving environment.
	Be mindful of the Carb Clock. Try to consume at least 60 percent of your daily calories by 5 P.M.; eliminate any starch after 5 P.M.
	Increase bulk and fiber with High-Quality/Low-Stress foods for sense of fullness throughout the day to successfully fight fat and carb cravings.
Physical activity	Energize yourself with forty-five minutes of cardiovascular physical activity each day. Get up and move and stretch for three to five minutes for every hour you sit. Strength-train with weights twice per week to maintain your muscle mass and thus boost your metabolism. For extra energy, take a walk outdoors and enjoy fresh air.
Restorative herbs	Use herbs to naturally activate and restore your chronically challenged stress system: peppermint, spearmint, vervain, skullcap, wild oat, St. John's wort, ginseng, rosemary, ginger, lemon balm, and cinnamon.

Box 10-3. **Rx for Stress Undereaters**

Goal	Maintain calm and sense of well-being.
	Objective: Avoid stress undereating throughout the day.
Calming attitude	Realize that food is not a negotiable item in your life, nor is it a daily torment. Let go of the rigid control you have over your eating behavior. Calm your perception of life stresses through the Relaxation Response or some form of meditation.
Calming eating	Avoid refined sugars.
	Stop skipping meals and try not to be food phobic.
	Plan to eat five small meals each day.
	Under stress try to eat at least part of your normal meals.
	Prioritize High-Quality/Low-Stress foods that include fruits and vegetables as well as high-fibered starches (brown bread, whole wheat pasta, brown rice).
	Focus on consuming balanced amounts of protein each day; e.g., low-fat cheese sticks, yogurt, smoothies, cottage cheese, fish, etc.
	Destress your eating by learning to enjoy each meal. Taste and savor each bite.
Physical activity	Energize, as well as find calm, with forty-five minutes of vigorous cardiovascular physical activity each day. Avoid overtraining. Augment your regular exercise routine with yoga and tai chi. Exercise outdoors for as much of your aerobic activity as possible to lessen your anxiety. Strength-train with weights twice a week to maintain your muscle mass and thus metabolism.
Restorative herbs	Use herbs to naturally calm and restore your chronically challenged stress system: skullcap, wild oats, wood betony, vervain, chamomile, St. John's wort, valerian.

Appendix A: Glossary

adrenal glands: two glands in the abdomen that, during the stress response, secrete adrenaline and cortisol

adrenaline: a chemical, often referred to as a neurotransmitter, produced and secreted by the adrenal glands during the stress response

Alarm Hormone: the master hormone of the stress response that triggers the body to handle the stress; also known as corticotropin-releasing hormone, or CRH, or a stress hormone.

Annoying But Livable (ABL) stress: stress that is integral to daily life, such as rush hour traffic

balanced caregiving: loving, nurturing, and caring for oneself as for others

beta-endorphin: a chemical secreted by the nervous system that provides pain relief as well as mood calming

cortisol: a hormone secreted by the adrenal gland as a response to stress; also known as glucocorticoid or stress hormone. Makes fuel available to cope with stress and induces appetite for refueling after stress.

CortiZone: the time of day (3 P.M. to midnight) when cortisol and adrenaline levels decrease in the bloodstream and individuals are at greatest risk for stress eating

Cushing's syndrome: a rare disease caused by a small tumor classically in the pituitary gland of the brain that causes prolonged exposure of body systems to high levels of cortisol

"fight-or-flight": the original way of describing how the body responds to stress by physical activity

health: the successful adaptation to life's stresses

homeostasis: the state of harmony or balance within the body

menopot: the fat around a woman's waistline that is above the abdominal muscle wall. This fat feels soft and can be grabbed easily. Also known as pinch an inch fat.

Metabolic Syndrome: a medical condition whose components include excessive intra-abdominal fat (Toxic Weight), diabetes, heart disease, high blood pressure, and possibly cancer. It is also known as Syndrome X.

Plan A: basic self-care done in one's unique living environment while stress is being managed

Plan B: basic self-care adjusted and done while under stress

regrouping: making transitions between Plan A and Plan B when stress disrupts one's normal healthy living routines

Relaxation Response: a form of meditation that neutralizes the stress response; first described by Dr. Herbert Benson

resilience: the ability to cope with life's stresses by being flexible and realistic and not resorting to self-destructive behaviors

reward system: a brain system that is triggered by the stress response to release a chemical, dopamine, that will allow an individual to perceive relief, pleasure, or reward when the stress is resolved

"stew and chew": the twenty-first-century response to stress; this response is to obsess and overeat rather than to fight or take flight as originally intended.

stress: the state of threatened homeostasis, or balance, in an individual

stress eating: the ingestion of food, primarily carbohydrates and fats, as a response to stress

Stress Fat: the fat depot inside the abdomen that is the natural source of fat fuel for the stress response; located below the abdominal muscle wall

stress hormones: include cortisol as well as Alarm Hormone

stressor: any person, place, or thing that threatens homeostasis, or balance, in an individual

Stress Overeater: an individual who overconsumes food under stress due to environmental factors as well as a probable genetic tendency to secrete inadequate amounts of Alarm Hormone when stressed

Stress-Resilient: an ability to cope with stress without resorting to self-destructive behaviors

stress response: the innate response of the mind and body to any stress

stress triggers: anything that makes an individual more vulnerable to triggering the stress response

Stress Undereater: an individual who eats less than normal amounts of food when under stress due to environmental factors as well as a probable genetic tendency to secrete higher than normal amounts of Alarm Hormone when stressed

Syndrome W: *w*omen, *w*orry, *w*eight, and *w*aist—an adaptation of the Metabolic Syndrome emphasizing women's unique tendencies that cause and result in the deposition of Toxic Weight

Toxic Stress: in the mind of an individual, a chronic, unrelenting stress that exposes body systems to prolonged, excessive levels of cortisol

Toxic Weight: excessive stress fat; an integral component of the Metabolic Syndrome. Associated with early disease and death from heart disease, diabetes, and probably cancer.

treading weight: maintaining one's body weight during stress

Appendix B: Additional Resources

Mind-Body

Online

American Psychological Association	helping.apa.org/mind_body
Ask Dr. Weil [Andrew Weil, M.D.]	www.drweil.com
Center for Anxiety & Stress Treatment	www.stressrelease.com
The Humor Potential, Inc. [Loretta LaRoche]	www.stressed.com
The Institute for Stress Management	www.hyperstress.com
International SPA Association	www.globalspaguide.com
The Life Sciences Institute of Mind-Body Health	www.healthy.net/univ/profess/schools/edu/lsi
Mental Health Resources [Lima Associates]	www.lima-associates.com
Mind/Body Medical Clinic at Beth Israel Deaconess Medical Center	mindbody.harvard.edu
National Center for Complementary and Alternative Medicine	nccam.nih.gov
National Institute of Mental Health	www.nimh.nih.gov
Omega Institute for Holistic Studies	omega-inst.org
Yoga Journal's Yoga Net	www.yogajournal.com

Organizations
American Psychological Association (APA)
750 First Street NE
Washington, DC 20002-4242
(202) 336-5500
publicinterest@apa.org

International SPA Association (ISPA)
546 East Main Street
Lexington, KY 40508
(888) 651-ISPA (4772)

Mind/Body Medical Clinic at Beth Israel Deaconess Medical Center
One Deaconess Road
Boston, MA 02215
(617) 632-9530; fax (617) 632-7383
mbclinic@caregroup.harvard.edu

National Center for Complementary and Alternative Medicine (NCCAM)
NCCAM Clearinghouse
P.O. Box 8218
Silver Spring, MD 20907-8218
(888) 644-6226; fax (301) 495-4957

National Institute of Mental Health (NIMH)
NIMH Public Inquiries
6001 Executive Boulevard
Room 8184, MSC 9663
Bethesda, MD 20892-9663
(301) 443-4513; fax (301) 443-4279
nimhinfo@nih.gov

Omega Institute for Holistic Studies
260 Lake Drive
Rhinebeck, NY 12572
(800) 944-1001
comments@omega-inst.org

Tools with Heart
A Woman's Book of Changes
15332 Antioch Street, Suite 459
Pacific Palisades, CA 90272
(888) 256-8762

Nutrition

Online

American Dietetic Association	www.eatright.org
American Heart Association	www.amhrt.org
American Society for Clinical Nutrition	www.faseb.org/ascn
Fitness Online [Home to Weider family magazines, including *Shape* and *Natural Health*]	www.fitnessonline.com
*on*health	onhealth.com
Shape Up America!	www.shapeup.org
Vegetarian Resource Group	www.vrg.org

Organizations

American Dietetic Association (ADA)
216 West Jackson Boulevard
Chicago, IL 60606-6995
(800) 877-1600; (312) 899-0040; fax (312) 899-4739
(800) 366-1655 (Consumer Hotline)
hotline@eatright.org; infocenter@eatright.org

American Heart Association (AHA)
National Center
7272 Greenville Avenue
Dallas, TX 75231
(800) AHA-USA1 (242-8721)
(888) MY-HEART (694-3278), Women's Health Information

American Society for Clinical Nutrition (ASCN)
9650 Rockville Pike
Bethesda, MD 20814-3998
(301) 530-7110; fax (301) 571-1863
secretar@acsn.faseb.org

Shape Up America!
6707 Democracy Boulevard
Suite 306
Bethesda, MD 20817
(301) 493-5368

Physical Activity

Online

American College of Sports Medicine   www.acsm.org

American Council on Exercise   www.acefitness.org

The Cooper Institute   www.cooperinst.org

FitnessLink   www.fitnesslink.com

The FitnessZone   www.fitnesszone.com

Shape Up America!   www.shapeup.org

Weider Publications   www.fitnessonline.com

Yoga Journal   www.yogajournal.com

Organizations

American College of Sports Medicine (ACSM)
P.O. Box 1440
Indianapolis, IN 46206-1440
(317) 637-9200

American Council on Exercise (ACE)
5820 Oberlin Drive, Suite 102
San Diego, CA 92121-3787
(619) 535-8227

Cooper Institute for Aerobics Research (CIAR)
12330 Preston Road
Dallas, TX 75230
(214) 701-8001

Shape Up America!
6707 Democracy Boulevard
Suite 306
Bethesda, MD 20817
(301) 493-5368

Appendix C: Rockport Fitness Walking Test

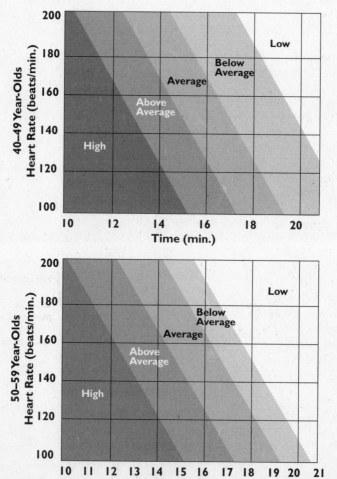

Appendix D: Major Muscle Groups

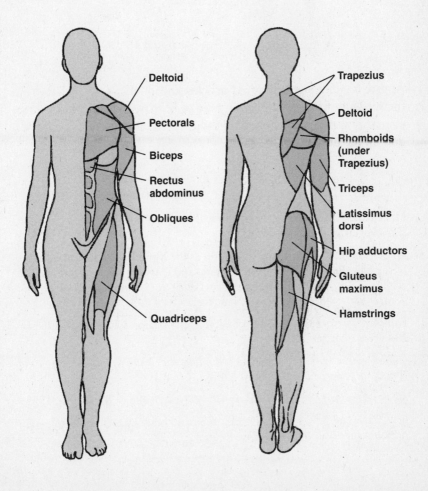

Front view labels:
- Deltoid
- Pectorals
- Biceps
- Rectus abdominus
- Obliques
- Quadriceps

Back view labels:
- Trapezius
- Deltoid
- Rhomboids (under Trapezius)
- Triceps
- Latissimus dorsi
- Hip adductors
- Gluteus maximus
- Hamstrings

Selected Bibliography

Approximately eight hundred articles and books were reviewed in the writing of this text. For the sake of brevity, I have included here primarily those publications that will be of most use and easiest to find by the nonscientist.

Stress/Mind-Body

H. Benson with M. Stark, *Timeless Healing: The Power and Biology of Belief* (New York: Scribner, 1996).

H. Benson, E.M. Stuart, and associates at the Mind/Body Medical Institute of the New England Deaconess Hospital and Harvard Medical School, *The Wellness Book: The Comprehensive Guide to Maintaining Health and Treating Stress-Related Illness* (New York: Carol Pub. Group, 1992).

P. Björntorp (1993), "Visceral obesity: a 'civilization syndrome,'" *Obesity Research* 1(1):206–222.

J. Borysenko with L. Rothstein, *Minding the Body, Mending the Mind* (Reading, MA: Addison-Wesley, 1987).

W. B. Cannon, *The Wisdom of the Body* (New York: W.W. Norton, 1932).

T. F. Cash and P. E. Henry (1995), "Women's body images: the results of a national survey in the USA," *Sex Roles* 33:19–28.

G. P. Chrousos and P. W. Gold (1992), "The concepts of stress and stress system disorders. Overview of physical and behavioral homeostasis," *Journal of the American Medical Association* 267(9):1244–1252.

———. (1998), "A healthy body in a healthy mind—and *vice versa*—the damaging power of 'uncontrollable' stress," *Journal of Clinical Endocrinology and Metabolism* 83(6):1842–1845.

G. P. Chrousos et al. eds., "Stress: basic mechanisms and clinical implications," *Annals of the New York Academy of Sciences,* v. 771 (New York: The New York Academy of Sciences, 1995).

G. P. Chrousos, D. J. Torpy, and P. W. Gold. (1998), "Interactions between the hypothalamic-pituitary-adrenal axis and the female reproductive system: clinical implications," *Annals of Internal Medicine* 129(3):229–240.

Dalai Lama, *Ethics for the New Millennium* (New York: Riverhead Books, 1999).

S. B. Heymsfield, et al. (1994), "Menopausal changes in body composition and energy expenditure," *Experimental Gerontology* 29(3–4):377–389.

J. K. Kiecolt-Glaser, et al. (1995), "Slowing of wound healing by psychological stress," *The Lancet* 346(8984):1194–1196.

L. LaRoche. *Relax—You May Only Have a Few Minutes Left: Using the Power of Humor to Overcome Stress in Your Life and Work* (New York: Villard, 1998).

K. R. Pelletier, *Sound Mind, Sound Body: A New Model for Lifelong Health* (New York: Simon & Schuster, 1994).

T. T. Perls, M. H. Silver with J. F. Lauerman, *Living to 100: Lessons in Living to Your Maximum Potential at Any Age* (New York: Basic Books, 1999).

J. O. Prochaska, J. C. Norcross, and C. C. DiClemente, *Changing for Good: The Revolutionary Program That Explains the Six Stages of Change and Teaches You How to Free Yourself From Bad Habits* (New York: William Morrow, 1994).

K. Räikkönen et al. (1999), "Anger, hostility, and visceral adipose tissue in healthy postmenopausal women," *Metabolism: Clinical and Experimental* 48(9):1146–1151.

S. Rechtschaffen, *Timeshifting: Creating More Time to Enjoy Your Life* (New York: Doubleday, 1996).

A. Ressler (1998), " 'A body to die for': eating disorders and body-image distortion in women," *International Journal of Fertility and Women's Medicine* 43(3):133–138.

R. Sapolsky (1999), "Stress and your shrinking brain," *Discover* 20(3): 116–122.

R. M. Sapolsky, *Why Zebras Don't Get Ulcers: A Guide to Stress, Stress-Related Diseases, and Coping* (New York: W. H. Freeman, 1994).

H. Seyle, *The Stress of Life,* rev. ed. (New York: McGraw-Hill, 1976).

———. *Stress Without Distress* (New York: NAL, 1974).

C. Warren and P. J. Cooper (1988), "Psychological effects of dieting," *British Journal of Clinical Psychology*/The British Psychological Society 27(Pt 3):269–270.

Nutrition

L. L. Bernardis and L. L. Bellinger (1981), "Further nutritional characterization of dorsomedial hypothalamic hypophagia in rats: diet consistency, finickiness, self-selection of diets, starvation and realimentation and 'stress eating,' " *Journal of Nutrition* 111(4):721–732.

J. Brand-Miller and K. Foster-Powell (1999), "Diets with a low glycemic index: from theory to practice," *Nutrition Today* 34(2):64–72.

The Food Guide Pyramid (1996), U.S. Department of Agriculture HG–252.

K. Foster-Powell and J. B. Miller (1995), "International tables of glycemic index," *American Journal of Clinical Nutrition* 62(4):871S–890S.

N. Geary (1998), "The effect of estrogen on appetite," Medscape Women's Health 3(6):3.

B. Healy, *A New Prescription for Women's Health: Getting the Best Medical Care in a Man's World* (New York: Viking, 1995).

A. L. Hirschberg (1998), "Hormonal regulation of appetite and food intake," *Annals of Medicine* 30(1):7–20.

Institute of Medicine, Division of Health Promotion and Disease Prevention, R. L. Berg and J. S. Cassells, eds., *The Second Fifty Years: Promoting Health and Preventing Disability* (Washington, D.C.: National Academy Press, 1990).

A. S. Levine and J. E. Morley (1981), "Stress-induced eating in rats," *American Journal of Physiology* 241(1):R72–R76.

M. D. Mifflin et al. (1990), "A new predictive equation for resting energy expenditure in healthy individuals," *American Journal of Clinical Nutrition* 51(2):241–247.

G. Oliver and J. Wardle (1999), "Perceived effects of stress on food choice," *Physiology & Behavior* 66(3):511–515.

E. Somer, *Food and Mood: The Complete Guide to Eating Well and Feeling Your Best* (New York: Holt, 1995).

Physical Activity

1996 Surgeon General's Report.

American College of Sports Medicine Position Stand (1998), "The recommended quantity and quality of exercise for developing and maintaining cardiorespiratory and muscular fitness, and flexibility in healthy adults," *Medicine and Science in Sports and Exercise* 30(6):975–991.

K. D. Brownell (1995), "Exercise and obesity treatment: psychological aspects," *International Journal of Obesity and Related Metabolic Disorders* 19 Suppl 4:S122–S125.

A. Byrne and D. G. Byrne (1993), "The effect of exercise on depression, anxiety and other mood states: a review," *Journal of Psychosomatic Research* 37(6):565–574.

L. D. Dugmore et al. (1999), "Changes in cardiorespiratory fitness, psychological wellbeing, quality of life, and vocational status following a 12 month cardiac exercise rehabilitation programme," *Heart* 81(4):359–366.

Healthy People 2000: National Health Promotion and Disease Prevention Objectives. DHHS Publication No. (PHS) 91-50213.

G. R. Hunter et al. (1998), "A role for high intensity exercise on energy balance and weight control," *International Journal of Obesity and Related Metabolic Disorders* 22(6):489–493.

F. Kronenberg (1994), "Hot flashes: phenomenology, quality of life, and search for treatment options," *Experimental Gerontology* 29(3–4):319–336.

L. H. Kushi et al. (1997), "Physical activity and mortality in postmenopausal women," *Journal of the American Medical Association* 277 (16):1287–1292.

M. E. Nelson with S. Wernick, *Strong Women Stay Slim* (New York: Bantam Books, 1998).

J. E. Manson et al. (1999), "A prospective study of walking as compared with vigorous exercise in the prevention of coronary heart disease in women," *New England Journal of Medicine* 341(9):650–658.

R. R. Pate et al. (1995), "Physical activity and public health. A recommendation from the Centers for Disease Control and Prevention and the American College of Sports Medicine," *Journal of the American Medical Association* 273(5):402–407.

A. S. Ryan et al. (1995), "Resistive training increases fat-free mass and maintains RMR despite weight loss in postmenopausal women," *Journal of Applied Physiology* 79(3):818–823.

L. Slaven and C. Lee (1997), "Mood and symptom reporting among middle-aged women: the relationship between menopausal status, hormone replacement therapy, and exercise participation," *Health Psychology* 16(3): 203–208.

R. I. Slupik ed., *American Medical Association Complete Guide to Women's Health* (New York: Random House, 1996).

P. Terry et al. (1999), "Lifestyle and endometrial cancer risk: a cohort study from the Swedish Twin Registry," *International Journal of Cancer* 82(1):38–42.

W. L. Westcott, *Strength Fitness,* 4th ed. (Dubuque, IA: William C. Brown Publishers, 1995).

T. P. White and the editors of the University of California at Berkeley Wellness Letter, *The Wellness Guide to Lifelong Fitness* (New York: Rebus, 1993).

W. C. Willett, W. H. Dietz and G. A. Colditz (1999), "Guidelines for healthy weight," *New England Journal of Medicine* 341(6):427–434.

Slides of CTs (page 29, 31)

P. M. Peeke and G. P. Chrousos (1995), "Hypercortisolism and obesity," *Annals of the New York Academy of Sciences* 77:665–676. With permission.

Index

Page numbers in *italics* refer to tables and figures.